FRAN MACILVEY

MAKING MIRACLES

FRAN MACILVEY
https://www.franmacilvey.com

Published by HEARTWELL PUBLISHING
© FRAN MACILVEY 2018

Cover design, typesetting and formatting: Jane Dixon-Smith

ISBN: 9781999713621 (paperback)
ISBN: 9781999713638 (ebook)

CONTENTS

ACKNOWLEDGEMENTS

I acknowledge the help of my small army of friends, my angels and guides for the writing of this small volume: I saw that it had been bound in a red cover long before I started.

I, the fiery light of divine wisdom
I ignite the beauty of the plains,
I sparkle the waters.
I burn the sun and the moon and the stars
With wisdom I order all rightly.
I adorn the earth.
I am the breeze that nurtures all things green.
I am the rain coming from the dew
That causes the grasses to laugh
with the joy of life.
I call forth tears, the aroma of holy work.
I am the yearning for good.

Hildegard of Bingen (1098–1179)

DISCLAIMER

The author of this book does not dispense medical advice or prescribe the use of any technique as a form of treatment for physical or medical problems without the advice of a physician, either directly or indirectly. The intention of the author is to offer information of a general nature to help you in your quest for emotional or spiritual well-being. In the event that you use any of the information in this book for yourself, the author and publisher assume no responsibility for your actions.

None of the suggestions included in this book is intended to replace the care of a physician or to interfere with a diagnosis, prescribed medicines or therapies. Each suggestion is based solely around the author's personal experiences and is never intended to substitute for existing care regimes.

The author writes from her own very personal experiences and reflections only, and as the outcome of her observations. Her personal beliefs are constantly evolving. Nothing she writes or has written is intended to detract from the value or worth of any other person's experiences, beliefs, faith or witness.

INTRODUCTION

As readers of my earlier work will know, I was born with cerebral palsy, the youngest child in a family of high achievers. In my infancy, life felt gilded with light and promise. As I grew older and my differences became almost impossible to ignore, life transmogrified into a decades-long struggle to fit in with other people's expectations, a hope doomed to failure. I longed to join in, but my sense of my oddities froze me to the spot. I could not easily take part in active games: I crawled and hobbled, then limped about on crutches, and I seemed to spend most of my time falling, and failing to keep up with other people. In the process of growing older and falling short in most comparisons I set up for myself, life lost its shine and I spent decades trying to recapture that sense of early optimism. At kindergarten, at school, at University and at work, I spent years rushing frantically to meet most of the "normal" expectations before the truth finally caught up with me: If you stop running, stop trying to keep up, perhaps you will discover there is an easier way to live.

When I was a child, my insecurities ran rampantly around me and I felt like "piggy in the middle". I habitually attempted the impossible – to climb high ladders, dance the cha-cha, skip for Britain...and failed miserably. It was never my homely, bookish achievements that I was proud of. Being able to write stories, laugh or listen? Who cared about these? I wanted to join in with the crowd who were skipping and playing hockey and basketball, but that was always going to be difficult so, after years of trying too hard at all the wrong things, I opted out. My passivity and resignation became increasingly marked with every year that passed.

Because the physical restrictions and "no-win" situations I have faced were so numerous, historically I responded by "choosing" to do nothing. I became a self-saboteur of the simplest things – like venturing outside – as well as my most exciting ideas. The pain of trying and failing was so intense, I found myself doing nothing for a very long time, many years.

But "sitting this one out" is, I realized rather late in the day, yet another no-win situation. While I have chosen to sit and wait and see, I have gained little, except perhaps a plethora of observed detail that might fit into a story which I might write sometime… as soon as I can get round to it.

I got past this entrenched swing from frantic (in) action – immersed in all the boring minutia that was expected of me – to inertia and depression by finally waking up to the personal cost to me and my family. Bored almost literally to death, I decided that walking my own path – taking that chance – had to feel better than all the grey, endless nothingness which was the backdrop of my usual expectations. Learning to listen to what I really wanted, and deciding to aim for that, didn't seem a risk as much as a life-saving necessity. I made up my mind, in effect, that I would rather take the chance of failing, than die inside a little more each day because I was afraid even to try.

There must have come a time when I first realised that I truly wanted to *live*; and that maybe writing would help me to find some answers. Having decid-ed, I must then have accepted the possibility that someone might get annoyed, someone would cut me off or hate me for being honest in what I wrote. These are the kinds of choices and decisions that most adolescents deal with; and here I am, admitting to not having had the courage to accept them until my early forties. By then, I finally understood that by not taking chances with my future, what might I lose? My health, all I held dear, the will to live…?

Spirit impelled me to leave my armchair, switch on my computer, sit down and start tapping away at my keyboard. They sent ideas, delight and energy, as well as more particular sensations of heat and light, pictures of colour and vivid flashes to awaken my memories. Theirs was a powerful challenge, a final throw of the dice. *Do this now, before you change your mind and get stuck once more in sitting still.*

Failure on my part to listen to soul promptings or guidance often leads to physical and emotional decline. To ensure that I stayed steady and completed the tasks I had started, Spirit, I see now, are always sending messages of reassurance. Increasingly, I know I am never alone and that my plans are being watched over. None of us is ever alone and we are watched with love, whatever we are doing.

IN THE BEGINNING

I have a notebook that usually sits by my bed. Within its pages and those of its predecessors, I have been recording pictures, dreams and understandings that have come to me down the years. It doesn't matter in the least where these ideas originate, since we all access personal wisdom in different ways. What matters is the outcome: an accumulation of insights and awareness that over time has enabled me to re-evaluate most of my beliefs and opinions, in a life-long process that ultimately empowers me to live more fully and with greater purpose.

In the course of my life I have weathered many challenges: disability, poverty, decades of depression and self-hatred, fear of loneliness and failure, emotional devastation; yet because much of that pain has been unconscious, I have not, until recently, seen the repeating nature of many of my difficulties: that an opportunity, for example, to be more gentle will keep returning to me until I can learn – at last! – that gentleness serves me as well as other people, my husband, my daughter, my mother and sisters. Gentleness has made my life more comfortable, just as learning to still the chatter in my head has made it more peaceful.

We can all think again about what we believe and how we are choosing to live, asking ourselves at intervals where we might like to see improvements. When we make any decision to change, progress is slow and uncertain. But help and insights are always available, so long as we can resist the urge to dismiss coincidences and chance occurrences when they do show up, even though they may not be easy to explain.

With this volume, I would like to share with you some of what I have discovered from gathering and paying attention to dreams, and how this process helps me to evolve new and more effective approaches to deal with life's challenges. Engaging with the guidance that we each receive, we cannot help but witness the power of miracles – chance encounters, inspirations, coincidences – playfully shaping our lives. All our dreams are unique; and naturally, our discoveries highlight individual challenges and solutions. Yet, whatever our particular hopes or circumstances, certain core messages are reliably consistent.

I am persuaded to begin now because my daughter is growing older. When she starts to ask those questions about Life, the Universe and Everything that we all ask – Why are we here? What is the point of life? Where did I leave my keys? – I would like at least to offer her the chance to take a free ride on some of my own mistakes and learning curves. Although nagging questions such as "Why?" tend to be answered for each of us by different twists and turns in the road, in what we see when our faces are cast in this or that direction, perhaps Seline will find something helpful in what is written here. She has helped me in countless ways, so maybe with this book I can begin to repay my debt to her.

It is my experience borne out every day, that miracles do not only belong to the old man on the hill who eats winkles from the seashore at low tide and contents himself with living a singular, solitary life doling out comforting platitudes to tired executives who, in deference to the old man's wisdom, pause to remove their shoes and ties at the end of a long trudge over a pitted coral shoreline. No-one, be they saint or rogue, is beyond the reach of chance events and encounters that have a potentially transformative effect. Indeed, one of their purposes is to remind us that appearances are deceptive: we have far more in common with each other than we realize.

Likewise, we make our lives needlessly difficult if we continue to believe that miracles, as we have been accustomed to reading about them, are confined to the Bible and other sacred texts, or if we cling doggedly to the view that the last time anyone encountered anything miraculous was when Jesus fed the five thousand with a handful of sprats and two small loaves of bread. Miracles wrap themselves around us all the time, existing and unfolding continuously in the here and now. Once we notice how they work as part of the benign process of our being alive, miraculous discoveries can happily inform everything we do.

Briefly, it is a matter of taking time to notice whatever is unfolding around us. First we notice, which helps us to believe. Then we begin to suspect what we think we already know. Once we know, we have the keys to the kingdom, even if, in this heavy, busy world we are apt to lose them from time to time. When we do, we can cheerfully ask the Locksmith in the Sky for another set, knowing s/he has a limitless supply.

We are always ready to begin again. We can refresh our resolve constantly. Picking ourselves up from our latest disappointments, we can smilingly re-engage with those nudges we get and with our lighter feelings which help us rediscover a path to take us forward. Spirit knows it is a heavy planet we live on and difficult. So why should we not look for help and accept solutions that offer themselves to us? Spirit loves to encourage us by sending us what we need, sometimes even before we know that we need it. Information, advice, even leaflets through the door might be invitations to consider something that Spirit can see coming our way, but which we, from our vantage point down here on Earth, have not yet noticed would be useful. All the time, life offers practical help and guidance, as well as fresh inspiration and encouragement, if we have the patience to listen, and the faith to act as we are led.

THE WORD WAS JOY

I toyed with naming my last book "Happiness Is Easy", which on reflection, made me uneasy. A title such as this suggests that happiness is trite, that it can be picked up with our groceries at the supermarket, along with the milk, fruit and vegetables or at the deli counter. More seriously, I am open to the accusation that I am making light of our everyday difficulties – I am being unkind, perhaps.

Then I understood. Like a dawning joy, the reply came to me. Happiness *is* easy and it *can* make light of our difficulties. Happiness reminds us that difficulties are placed before us so that, in rediscovering afresh how setbacks can be overcome, we remember our strength, flex our muscles and enjoy our power to deliberately create more positive outcomes. Throughout this whole life process that shows us how we can grow, we can become stronger. It sounds crazy, doesn't it? Yet, among the biggest challenges we face are not "our problems" but how we deal with them.

"The problem" may be that I am an impatient woman. So I may ask Life for help to be more patient, to be more understanding or more compassionate. Since I believe that all our requests are heard and answered, I may be sent fresh energy to help me cope, a little light healing, a nudge to do something that will refresh me, maybe a sprinkling of inspirational dreams. A different perspective may be revealed, so that I wake from a night's rest reminded of how lucky I am. All these things are re-energizing and increase my patience threshold.

Lessons may come along in a more practical way, too. If I ask for more patience, along with all the support I may hope to receive such an extra dash of optimism, space to make decisions or unexpected gifts coming my way, I may receive other practical help – lessons. My computer may not work or may go slow for days at a time. I may lose my keys or forget to take out the rubbish and have to return to retrieve it from the house when I am halfway down the street running to an appointment for which I am already late. I may encounter long queues in traffic or delays at the post-office. I wait for ages to be served while everyone else seems to receive immediate attention. My pay is overdue arriving in my account. Something valuable may get lost, or my daughter may have a problem that takes a lot of time to resolve. That all these things happen to me may not be because I am having a "truly awful day", though it probably feels like that at the time. Hold-ups which spark my impatience may be the answer to my prayers.

Because I have sincerely asked to be more patient, perhaps my prayer is being answered in a most practical way: difficulties or delays which would usually have me tearing my hair out with frustration will eventually have the desired effect. Through dealing with difficulties, I learn that it is better for me, easier, far more relaxing and effective if I try to accept every situation as it is and stop worrying about how it may turn out. I stop trying to push water uphill and so by slow degrees I learn that results work out better when I can act patiently and reserve judgement.

Having read hundreds of books about personal motivation, why things are as they are, and what existence means, theories about our purpose and meaning remain the compulsion of a lifetime. But, unfortunately for me, I seem to absorb lessons best when my life deals out a few practical home truths. After whole seasons of lessons and more lessons, finally I am learning that everything turns out better when I deliberately focus on staying relaxed and dwelling in whatever joy each situation contains. Indeed, "the problem" is not the circumstances we face, but how we handle them.

Understanding how this process – of awareness, request, application and renewed understanding –

can work for us is the real quantum leap, as we find reasons to stay with and benefit from all the bumpy nuts and bolts of our lives and what these ultimately can teach us.

We take such pains over our problems which in many ways we love to glorify, constantly reminding ourselves how challenging everything is, as if our adversity is a badge of honour. What if instead, we choose to use our personal strength more creatively? Before we leap off the deep end and start thrashing about in our grievances, we can stop, regroup and say, "Okay, so I have some problems. But what can I do right now, to feel better?" I suspect that what we really desire is the strength to react with the same centred acceptance whatever life throws our way.

The Universe rejoices in our calmness and in our peaceful happiness. When our lights shine and hum with contentment, I can just imagine how Life heaves a sigh of relief – "Thank goodness someone is still happy out there!" There is genuine delight in the sight of us gently busy, a source of love, calmly getting on with our lives and helping each other.

Miracles are one way in which Life reminds us that we are connected forever to the great expanse of Wholeness which displays qualities of total Love, Acceptance, Peace, Joy and Certainty. Though a process of rediscovery may feel by turns painful or blissful, there is nothing magical in arriving at an understanding that God – which we may call Source, the Universe, the Light, Life, Love, Yahweh, The Boss – rejoices with us when we recognize our connection with the Love that encompasses all things, feelings and states of being. If the limping man who walks again will call that a miracle, so be it.

Miracles ultimately remind us of our partnership and unity with Source. All of life moves in rhythms of togetherness and co-operation. Even as life forces may give the appearance of pulling apart, or falling to pieces, that process is part of the ultimate unity that reveals itself in growth, reconfiguration, healing and expansion. Natural systems depend utterly on mutual relationships in which it can be hard to see where one aspect stops and another starts. Mutually beneficial systems weave incredibly complex and beautiful webs.

We do not stand apart from beauty. We are part of the web. If loving impulses guide our actions, inevitably we inch towards wholeness, which is what we are all aiming for. Even when we do something that appears to place us at a disadvantage – like letting a queue of cars go in front of us, so that we add to our travel time or are late for an appointment – whenever our impulse springs from generosity or love, the outcome will *always* be beneficial for us. Making a worthwhile present and a future to look forward to, replete with the satisfaction of completion, is our ultimate purpose, though most of the time we are not consciously aware of this.

We can't live at elevated levels of consciousness all the time. Indeed, learning to live in the present is a constant daily discipline. Even so, our smallest agreement with new hope and with infinite possibilities for renewal helps us, by lifting away feelings of isolation, or the stress we sometimes feel when we dwell on our difficulties and aloneness. We are never meant to feel lonely, which is why we find negative states hard to live with and ruinous to our health. Isolation and negativity pull us down, away from higher, lighter truths which, when we remember them, remind us of our connectedness with each other.

It seems to me that when we ponder the making of miracles, we are considering a state of being in which our bits and pieces of worry, upset or insecurity no longer rule us, but are smoothed away with love and ultimately set aside. When we understand that, we know we are safe, since love is always with us, faithfully keeping us company while we mis-step on the bumpy highways and side-tracks of life. We will all reach our destinations eventually.

Our negative feelings and all the "bad" things that happen can serve a useful purpose. I argue, "Yes, I know you would like me to learn and I realise that I am being shown something important here but why does this all have to be so HARD?" I get upset that life seems to become easier one minute and then ten times harder the next. But setbacks, and the whole backwash of negative feelings that these produce, reveal our weaknesses and limits as well as our personal and moral boundaries. They help us to accept the need for rest; they teach us the joy of asking clearly for what we want and accepting help; they strengthen us by degrees, to stand up straight in the face of discouragement, criticism or confusion and clarify what we do and don't accept: all of which are very useful outcomes.

Uncomfortable feelings, if we can stand back and observe them instead of getting carried away by them, can be extremely enlightening. Shades of light and darkness illuminate our strengths and failings, allowing us to choose "what now?" By choosing, we determine what we stand for.

Am I doing what I desire? Perhaps my stomach is trying to ask me: will I be happy if I do this? If my stomach or my heart remain unmoved or are filled with cold, miserable feelings, the answer is a definite No; and if my body feels warm, vibrant and excited, the answer is a definite Yes.

When we are truly happy, we are following the path set for us by our soul, which acts in love and with infinite compassion. Since our soul cannot sit and chat with us companionably over a cup of tea, it uses feelings and emotions, as well as vivid dreams and coincidences, to continually communicate with us and help us stay on the most rewarding path to our next goals.

Where spiritual learning is concerned, I am impatient. I read voraciously, like to understand a topic quickly, and am always pushing on to the next great discovery. My mind leaps about like a frog in a race to reach the next pond, that bigger one over there. Not this one I am presently sitting in. It is difficult for me to be still. Yet, observation continually reminds me that whether I like it or not, progress towards peace and serenity is not linear, predictable or evenly spaced. Unfortunately, insights cannot be booked in advance, plugged in or programmed to turn up for us according to our stated preferences, say between nine and ten on a Sunday morning.

So it can be a challenge to contain any sparkling, bubbling impulses long enough to write a book about miracles and the colourful pictures and dreams that so often illuminate our higher purposes. To pin down "miracles" with lines drawn about by words may seem contrived. Perhaps we should give up the attempt before we are lost: the difference between a miracle experienced and the attempt to describe it is like trying to tell a friend about an amazing dream I had last night while she is turned away from me, listening to music on her MP3 player and we are separated by a thick pane of glass.

I cannot really *explain* to you how miracles happen. That is not how they reveal themselves. I *can* ask, what are your priorities? Do you want to be happier? Would you like to notice miracles near you today? If you answer a heartfelt yes, then you have found your best reason to begin and the only one you need. Our willingness, our impatience for change, is where we all start and what we build on. We can each discover new ways to make our experience of miracles more likely, more familiar and more welcome. Like waves breaking gently on a beach, small revelations meet our everyday lives haphazardly, with seeming carelessness, apparently by accident: it is not when I am *trying* to do a thing that it turns out best.

Occasionally, a stunning new perspective may rear up and "hit" us with a vividness and excitement that we can almost taste. Eureka moments can jolt us and open the door to a whole new way of seeing things. However, it is more likely that, like little daisies turning their heads to the light, or like small fawns turning their eyes calmly in our direction to explore, comprehension dawns slowly and gently, so that before we realize what is happening, we find ourselves smiling and hopeful again.

SOUL SPEAKS

Here is one of the first pieces I wrote. Its impact was so visceral that I was finally compelled to start a proper, organised dream journal and to persevere with it, despite my usual lazy tendencies. As anyone who knows me will tell you, getting me to persist with anything is itself a miracle, but with this I had little choice. Ignoring this sequence would have been like ignoring a truck hurtling towards me.

> I had a ghastly dream recently – a snapshot; a very colourful and extremely vivid nightmare; a single bright picture demanding to be noticed, its meaning not fully understood until the writing of it.
>
> I'm in a very small toilet room – yuck! – and the toilet bowl is padded; so it is quite hard, almost impossible, to dispose cleanly of urine that I am pouring away from lots of half-empty glass jars into the toilet. When I do aim for the pan a lot does hit the bottom,

where it is supposed to go; but a lot gets soaked into padding which lines the toilet bowl. The room is painted a deep blood red and is very claustrophobic, with barely space to turn around. A shelf, which someone has put up on three sides, runs around the room at shoulder height and further restricts my space to move; jars of urine are stacked about three high on the shelf all round me. In my face. Too much for me to handle.

I have one elbow up to keep the jars from sliding off the shelf; I have another hand not very successfully tipping out the contents down the toilet. Next to the shelf on the wall, someone has hung up a white wire basket, like an old- fashioned vegetable rack. It is fastened precariously, hanging on by one nail. Though the rack is hanging at a slant, only just holding, it is also stacked with pots and pans, piled high. I take the lid off one of the pots and I see a pair of hands tied at the wrists with strong white string, looking almost like a bouquet garni. So, my hands are tied, I am on the rack, somehow and my career is going down the pan. A gruesome dream, deeply disturbing but memorable.

According to my personal lexicon, this dream was telling me that I must take immediate, urgent action to change my employment, which my soul was forcefully reminding me was impossible and unrewarding: what do toilets and urine say about the type of work I was doing? What can anyone do, whose hands are tied and who has no private room to manoeuvre? The small, closeted space screams claustrophobia and the colours are dark, blood red, intimate, womb-like. The odds are stacked against me. In other words: GET OUT OF THERE.

Compare that with the following waking experience, which I include here because it came to me shortly after I finally did get out of there and for the contrast it offers. Though not a dream, the following sequence had a great impact on me because, for the very first time, I actually noticed that Someone was trying to tell me something. I had started Listening.

At our holiday hotel

I have eaten the seeds of the pomegranate
– sweet and strong on the outside, powdery
and clinging on the inside. Seeds, pips
of patience, endurance, insight, courage,
wisdom. The taste lingers. I have received
many blessings and gifts, yet I have not
used them. I have received love, fair looks

and taste, intelligence, humour and luck, this last obvious from my having obtained all the former blessings. Yet for some reason I have lived a penumbral, peripheral life, refusing almost to breathe fully; to talk firmly or walk calmly. Why? Do I feel my living is a waste of space that could be better taken up by someone else? My midlife is almost upon me. The fresh, youthful spring has left my step and I crave now to fill more gently and fully the space cast by my shadow in the sun.

I am not a living regret or a disgrace. I need not beg for room to move over the green lawn of my life. I may now finally receive all the goods and gifts which life sees fit to bequeath to me, unselfishly and quietly filling a space.

Out of the dining-room bay window I saw a single tree and I said to myself without thinking, "That is me." On reflection, I considered this true: tall and frail, with pale dusky pink leaves, wistful, yet wishing to be more flamboyant. Supported on a pale, twisted line of a trunk, slender and leaning to one side, many-stemmed and insubstantial.

By contrast, through the same window, to one side I noticed many heavy, branching conifers closely set, marching in serried, organized ranks, uniform and indistinguishable. The other tree stood alone and several meters apart, pink, on a lawn of green, at once singular, elegant and sad. I considered all this in passing. The image I made of this reflected well my wish to be "like them". I acknowledged, also, that I could never be. I am a different tree with no solid brown trunk, not even green like the rest.

But Life took a further hand in my enlightenment, for I glanced by chance out of the adjacent window set neatly alongside the first. I saw in the second a glorious profusion of pink-leafed trees, with one or two edges, only, of green. Here there was no question that pink smiled broadly. It was no matter that there were several different shades. The contrast swept over me like sunshine and lightened my awareness like an omen: sudden, brilliant and sharp.

So clear and informed, so simple.

In dreams, symbolism is everything. There was so much that the Universe was telling me here: that I was ungrounded: I identified with a tree anchoring itself in the ground by several thin, twisting stems, not with the broad, strong trunk usually associated with trees. I am a dreamy, impractical type given to flights of fancy, like that sweet, singular tree. I would never fit in to the serried ranks of disciplined conifers that seemed to crowd around me. I was alone, lonely. But looking at the scene from a different perspective – out of an adjacent window – I saw lots of trees – people – like me! It seemed suddenly obvious: with a small change of perspective, many of my understandings would alter immediately. The optimism that leapt up then has stayed with me as a reassurance of better things to come.

ABOUT JOY

I am writing this book because I am inspired to: my fingers itch and ideas are popping into my head from all over the place. I cannot wait to discover how we make miracles. What are they? How do they work? Most importantly, can they work for me? Can I have them in my life every day?

Somehow, I hold a smiling memory that knows that we all can; but, rather like the tipster who hedges his bets and will only set up in business when he has worked out a fool-proof betting system, I wander unaware past the small signs that link my life with Universal laws which would, if I heeded them, make living so much easier and more rewarding. Truths wait quietly, overlooked, yet always hoping to be re-discovered. "This Way" says the marker, lost among overgrown bushes, which obscure the path where I once wandered easily and without a care. What memories can I summon now? Which path should I take?

How we find miracles in our lives is potentially such a high, grand subject that I could easily get carried away. Perhaps I could begin simply, with a few statements of "the obvious".

The practice of cultivating miracles begins not when we plan our day by saying, "Now let me see, this morning I am going over that mountaintop there to search for the magic at the end of that rainbow," nor if we decide we have to fast for a day or two, or even six months or six years to get in the mood. That is certainly not required, which is just as well. How many of us can afford the time or resources to search out the pristine wilderness that we seem to believe is so vital for our spiritual cleansing? Should only the well-heeled be entitled to miraculous assistance? The truth is far more straightforward.

We can begin right here, where we are now. We are invited to use as our starting point the thousand-and-one sights and happenings we encounter each day and which we mostly forget to notice. We can begin little by little to re-examine what might turn out to be enjoyable lessons hidden within our daily experiences.

It proves rewarding to re-examine the multitude of circumstances in my life that I usually take for granted and which I assume I must learn to tolerate, whether I like them or not. It may be that, as I make my way home on a Friday evening, I decide now would be a great time to make a start. Why wait? As soon as I get through the front door, I drop my bag, lift off my heavy work suit and kick off my shoes. While changing into my weekend gear, a deep sigh of relief escapes my obedient and well-controlled exterior. This is already something different. It dawns on me as I contemplate the delicious weekend ahead that I feel lighter and more playful. I like that feeling and so I ask quietly, "What do I really want to do this evening?" The question drifts over my head as I sit peacefully. Silently, an answer arrives beside me: "To rest in stillness."

Responding to our willingness to look again at Life and observe it differently, gentleness, hope and love reveal their faces, at first shyly and then with increasing joy and boldness, bursting open like fragrant tropical blossoms at the end of the long rains.

Without needing to know why or how, by being willing to watch and wait, we have already started a shift in our attitudes that will affect all our choices and relationships. Unfamiliar feelings of being more relaxed, more certain and more peaceful can, if we allow them, become our lifelong companions. Having walked alongside us from birth, the fragrant truth finally embraces us that if we choose, we may finally end our heavy dialogue with worry, pessimism, sorrow and failure.

Consider any of the following suggestions as an opening which you can pick up, examine at your leisure and put down again as you please. Each idea can be a tool, a "crow bar" to lever off some of the layers of expectation and "busyness" that pull us away from our centre of lightness. Which suggestion appeals to you, depends on how you feel about it. If any of them makes you uncomfortable or angry, ponder why that might be.

Slow Down

If we wish to notice loveliness we can begin by slowing down. Time and again I hear this story, or a version of it: "I was walking along the street when I suddenly noticed this beautiful bird flying low; I saw a beautiful moon rising over the horizon; I had to *slow down and take a picture of it* on my iPhone. I just had to!"

I suspect that we inhabit parallel spheres. Out there, up over our heads, one world spins beauty and magic all around us. Miracles hang suspended in time, waiting for us to see them. Down here, we do not usually observe anything special, so snugly are we fitted into our everyday "must do" lives.

Because we are so preoccupied with mind-centred tasks, we do not usually make much room in our day-to-day for the unexpected, though we could, quite easily. Isn't it easy for us to wait a moment, peaceful, before we rise from our beds in the morning? Are we able to let drop the worries of the day when we retire for the night? Whenever we pause for a moment, depth and colour begin to seep in around the edges of our thoughts, which are usually moving so quickly that they have very few occasions to pause, relax and expand. A clear intention to slow down allows us to step aside from our usual framework and from internal dialogues that tell us what we should be thinking and doing next.

What exciting possibilities are waiting to be rediscovered? By far the easiest way to see glimpses of this intoxicating, colourful life is to slow ourselves down. Did I say colourful? I hope so…

Colour Life In

What vividness is there in the stuff of our everyday lives? What brightness do we embrace? As we run about "thinking" and "doing" we seem to be plugged into an existence which is barely sketched in hurried outlines and which passes us by in a variety of muted greys or dark greens with occasional glimpses of metallic silver or red, like a long queue of cars ahead of us in a traffic jam. I don't suppose we pause to consider how much our usual pale colour scheme is at odds with what is lingering sweetly in the park. We are so busy that we don't even have time to think in colours. What a pity! Colours are part of life. If our minds are skipping so that we don't see any, we are certainly moving too quickly. Unsurprisingly, without colour, our lives may feel washed out or lacking energy.

In the parallel world that moves around us, a world which we try to pretend does not exist and that we dismiss as disorganized, untidy or chaotic, colours are everywhere. In the realm of miracles, colours rest quietly, perfectly at home, dancing and shimmering in everything and hoping to be noticed. It is deep beauty that we are letting ourselves in for, when we slow down and contemplate delight.

Next time you are on lunch break, I challenge you to go for a walk. Not along the corridor to the coffee machine or the accounts department. Not to your line manager to exchange views about the month's projected outcomes. Take yourself outside, somewhere you don't usually go. Make it part of your plan to count how many colours you spot and to notice how, in pausing to count colours, you amble, instead of marching purposefully. How many birds can you hear singing in the trees around you? Do you feel ease and gratitude for the change of scene? Does your breathing slow down? The energy we collect while walking also reminds us that there is no hurry. Even with five or ten minutes to spare, make it a new priority to rediscover the joy of lingering, sauntering, savouring your space and breathing deeply.

Embrace Silence

Many of us, probably most of us, have strong internal messages that school us into doing this job, deciding to finish this task to get on with that next thing. Old voices we listen to, tinged with negativity, like to remind us of our hard luck ("I always end up doing the boring jobs...", "I have to go to the office this weekend", "I hate getting stuck listening to this person", "I am so sick of waiting in traffic") or keep us in the grip of our usual routines and circuits.

Paying heed to internal voices – which are so often discouraging – does not help us to get jobs done. Sparky thoughts, sudden reminders are great; internal worry or guilt circuits are less useful. The thought and time we invest listening to our internal dialogues, constructing our justifications and retorts, distracts and drains our focus and energy. In paying such close attention to the constant flow of chatter, we forget that each job, no matter how mundane or repetitive, contains elements of novelty and enjoyment. In the stillness of the present, we can introduce humour, laughter and music. Even when we are unhappy, there is much we can improve, when we allow ourselves some stillness.

I don't suggest that you should never speak to your friends or join a silent community. However, I know that especially when doing jobs I find routine or dull, indulging in negative talk or listening to my usual weary head chatter makes my daily tasks a great deal harder, drawn out and tedious.

Embracing peace in the present, every facet of every situation reveals itself afresh from a closer, more intimate perspective. Silence invites simple solutions and gives us unexpected room to manoeuvre. Without a great deal of hard work or conscious effort, peace allows answers and the joy of the creative process to surface and come to our aid.

Ask

If we have the courage to slow down – even a little; and colour our lives in – just a bit; when we wait quietly for a moment, we automatically create more space and time. In that space it is helpful to remember that it is rude to push and shove, to expect and take ungraciously. Any sense of our entitlement which speaks of wanting, demanding, neediness or yearning is usually unproductive: the negativity in these attitudes repels gentle solutions.

If there is something we would truly like to have, it is more polite to ask and to go looking for it with a peaceful determination. If we desire something, or are looking for a solution to a problem, asking clearly and honestly for what we would like assists the process to work in our favour. We can address our requests to God, to Life, to our guardian angels, to our favourite tree, to that Entity we might think of as our Boss in the Sky or Dave, the Universal Organizer. If like me, you have historically found asking for help almost impossible, it does get easier with practice.

I ask once and immediately find it easier to ask again. I ask again and the next question waiting in the queue comes fast to my side. If we have never asked for help before, we may uncover hundreds of secret requests that we never dared to share suddenly begging to be released. Go ahead! You too can ask for anything you like and soon you will feel like a child in a sweet shop. It is perfectly acceptable to ask, any time you wish. And there is no difference in this circumstance between a small ask ("please can you get me a parking space?") and what we would see as a really big ask ("I would love a new home"). Not all our requests will be met immediately – imagine if they were! – and there are many reasons for this. But clearly asking for what we wish is a good place to start.

I now ask for help when I would like to make a meal quickly, when I would like a store cupboard ingredient, when I would like to start work on time, when I need to stop and rest, when I am securing my home for the night, when I would like to sleep well, when I am hoping for good weather, when I would like more energy or to release negative feelings, when I'm searching for a perfect book, when I need a parking space or a bus or taxi, when I have forgotten to telephone my friend. Help is available for all our small requests as well as our grand projects.

It feels truly liberating to put down the armour of self-reliance and joyfully whisper for whatever it is we would like. Once we have asked, we can let the question go. Almost without our noticing, results come to us.

If we were able to reach that level of completely faithful bliss which simply knows that all our wishes are granted, we would find that we no longer needed to make any requests or even say prayers, since Life would already be anticipating perfectly whatever we wish for. All our prayers would become valuable opportunities to offer thanks and gratitude for our blessings: "Thank you for all the joy you have given me: I create with deliberate, joyful intention, knowing that what we are doing and planning together is wonderful. I trust that everything is unfolding for my best and that you have my life well in hand. From your lofty perch you can see much farther into my future than I ever can. I trust you to guide me easily and happily to my best outcomes. I know that, because you love me, everything works out perfectly for me."

A level of faith which *knows* that all our prayers are always answered and that everything is constantly ordered for our best interests has only been attained by a handful of spiritual masters. It is easier for the rest of us, if we realize that there is no shame in asking for help whenever we wish. The answers we receive are often surprising and delightful.

Surrender

When we consciously begin to slow down, sooner or later another feeling will creep up and quietly tap us on the shoulder. Once we begin the delightful process of opening out our sense of wonder and giving it space to breathe, when we enjoy watching sunlight playing in the ripples on the water, or late afternoon shadows flitting teasingly over the path in front of us, sooner or later we will find ourselves rejoicing that we are part of the miracle. Then, perhaps, will come a quiet feeling of surrender. You may call it acceptance or letting go. However you might experience that sense of release, the outcome is the same: we stop watching, counting and being so careful. We Surrender to What Is.

Surrendering means we stop trying to fix everything the way we *think* it ought to be. Surrendering to what is, allows all the defences we have built up and cling to their freedom to collapse, to flow away and dissolve, allowing us to see life anew and accept what we see and feel without trying to mend, sort or even understand it. We rediscover an apparent contradiction that I take great delight in: accepting the world as it is without trying to understand it allows endless ideas and amusing solutions to float quietly up towards us with the minimum of fuss and effort. Thus, we see very simply what we can do now, without engaging our mental processes in endless worrisome internal dialogues with our many options or with "what might go wrong".

Surrender ultimately means handing over every concern in our lives and agreeing that we do not want or need to hold on to or retain ownership of any heaviness that comes from being preoccupied, feeling alone, burdened or tired. Surrendering is effectively an invitation to Life to take care of the details for us, please, while we content ourselves with making decisions and choices that uplift us right now – decisions that make us feel powerful – and help us to express more fully *who we are*. With surrender comes increasing peace and freedom to make choices effectively and to watch them unfolding. When we release our burdens and leave our minds in peace, rejoicing in the knowledge that there is much we do not understand, miracles flow towards us.

THE POWER OF UNIVERSAL CREATION

In whatever way we perceive the power that animates Life, Source seems to me to include all Life, total Love, Light, ultimate Peace, total Acceptance or All That Is. Source, as well as being the power that creates, encompasses everything. I may name that power Life, Source, Spirit, God, Creator and Love; and to me these terms are synonymous.

It is said that Source knows everything. Yet mere "knowing" is not entirely satisfying. Like us, Source also wants to know what "everything" *feels like*. To know something intellectually is not the same as experiencing it at first hand, as we can all appreciate. When we ask, "Can I see that?" do we not pick objects up into our hands all the better to examine them, feel their shapes, contours and weight? The exploration of life is so much more interesting when we add the depth of touch and feeling, instead of merely looking or reading about stuff in a magazine.

I find it most helps me to work within an understanding that all forms of life are different facets of (the whole of) Life. From the original Whole, all living creatures have been created in all kinds and forms, in order for them to experience what it feels like to live and be themselves. Since we originate from Source, we are part of and therefore always connected to Source, though we aren't often aware of our deep connection. Love inhabits our skin and enjoys feeling that part of God-self that is you or me, or that flower over there, that white star or that dark stream. So it follows that nothing on Earth needs to justify its existence by *doing* anything. That any part of God's Life simply celebrates existence by being itself is enough.

Having created life in all its forms, and through the ongoing cycle of continual re-creation, Source Which Is Everything experiences the joy of all the differing parts of creation as well as the total joy inherent in the whole.

If we want to do more than just be, of course we can. Life would be pretty uninspiring if we all lazed around being spacey. One of the strongest urges in the natural world, if not the strongest, is for re-creation. What Life creates – birds, bees, all of us, the Universe and everything – exists to mimic its creator, by creating something by and of itself.

We can choose what we create from the many

choices that are available to us: the good, the bad, the indifferent, the annoying. Within our creativity lie our unique routes to a new sight of life. Depending on what we create, we may see life more darkly, or from a lighter, more fulfilling perspective. As naturally as water flows, we are constantly in the midst of our personal, unique creative movement.

We allow our choices to be dictated by the choices or beliefs of the wider community. When that prevalent mind-set is pessimistic or unhelpful (when the common mind-set is that *life is a drag and the world is heading for disaster*) it can be a huge challenge to see past negative messages such as these and focus on what we would prefer to make manifest instead.

Individually and collectively, we are always creating something; and by and large, we all wish for the same outcomes: for love, for peace, good health, meaningful work and personal satisfaction, material wealth, and happiness. Human preferences and purposes are refined through every activity we undertake: through thinking delicious thoughts, deciding what we are going to do now, deciding how we wish to respond to a given set of circumstances – or indeed, whether we will react at all – selecting a new pair of shoes, baking biscuits, choosing to accept every situation as it is, phoning our friends or doing nothing much today after all. Even while we are sitting still, we are creating *something* with our thoughts, feelings and beliefs. However hard we may push that power away, deny it or cull it back out of sight, the flow of our choices is constantly finding outlets. Creative power is as inevitable as breathing.

Time and space are part of the framework within which we can see our choices playing out. So instead of drifting aimlessly or blaming others for where we find ourselves, don't you think it would be a good idea to change our minds and step forward with deliberate intent? If we take a few wrong turns on the way or decide to set a different course, instead of seeing our "mistakes" as problematic, we can agree with a grin, "*This* is what I prefer to do – not that – because this feels more joyful and my life feels more meaningful when I go this way."

We have a very significant part to play. With an expanded awareness, we may notice the impact of even our smallest choices on our lives and on the lives of family, friends, colleagues and people we will never meet. Understanding that we are powerful, whatever we may be doing, we feel increasingly empowered to choose those creative impulses that Feel Good. Shall I use my power positively now? Or shall I ignore it, or worse, focus on what is "wrong" in my life and wallow in my misfortune? Shall I hurt myself today, or have fun? Shall I laugh now or cry? What makes me feel good…?

When we appreciate our innate power to ask for help in creating the life of our dreams; when we slow down and colour life in; when we surrender and allow Life to help us find answers, we rejoin – at least for some of the time – the magical world of Light that creeps around our everyday edges, reminding us of the joy waiting peacefully to reconnect with us.

PLAYING OUR PART IN THE GAME

Throughout countless Universes the power of Life has been and is constantly creating, expanding and manifesting outcomes. That the Laws of Life unfold as they do, consistently, whether we are young or old, tired or energized and filled with hope or despair, should give us cause to relax and celebrate: we can feel optimistic, overflowing with feelings of love and self-worth; we can be self-critical, painfully shy or depressed. Whatever our situation, the many laws that govern the workings of the world are unchanging, though they challenge, change and remake us, constantly. Their very constancy and reliability is the key to understanding how we can work with them to improve our lives. In the following chapters I touch on four universal laws which have shown me new ways to understand how the world works: free will, cause and effect, the law of attraction and the law of reflection. I suspect that whatever we call these processes and however we see them working, we are all familiar with them at some level.

That the Laws of Life are so inexorably impartial might seem unfair. You might wonder, "How come no-one sees how hard I work? I have prayed so long for change, for improvements, yet no-one is listening. Here I am, still stuck in this lousy house, in this terrible relationship, with a no-hope job. When will life get better for me?" It is so true, that in a state of anxiety or hopelessness, it is difficult to see our lives transforming into anything positive.

Creative power is inherent. In that sense, there is nothing we can do about it. Every time we sit, move, believe, breathe, ponder, decide, or speak, we are in a creative flow that takes us in this direction or that, towards this goal or away from that path. In every second we are choosing. Our highest beliefs about ourselves, such as, "I am lovable and I deserve to be happy", "I deserve peace in my life", "The Universe supports me with Love" and "Divine timing is always perfect", are constantly unfolding consequences which can, if we allow them to, empower us to become more than we ever dreamed possible. And since most of us are here for many years, we will find it rewarding to think and do the best we can, with whatever tools and gifts are available to us now.

Universal laws which govern the way the world works (such as cause and effect and the law of attraction) unfold with relentless inevitability, informing and shaping all our individual creative choices. When we first consciously deploy them – presumably in the hope of improving our lives – we probably do so haltingly, as when we first learned to walk. We may have fallen or stumbled thousands of times when we were toddlers, but we never stopped trying, did we? We wanted to get up, move faster and discover exciting new things higher up. In the same way, as our awareness expands, the creative powers that underpin the Universe continually urge us forward in a process which constantly widens and lifts our perspectives.

For example, I might see myself as a successful business person. I am industrious and diligent, influential and learned; and what I contribute to my organization is recognized and rewarded handsomely. I am happy and successful. Then one day, I feel dissatisfied. I wonder what else there is to do, apart from putting in a hundred hours a week and seeing the kids every second weekend. As I leave the building, I see a homeless person begging in the street. He doesn't look like my usual idea of a drop-out. He has short hair, a clear complexion and a great smile. So I stop and listen. He tells me he has recently been asked to leave the family home, because he doesn't get on with his mother's new partner. He is shivering and his clothes are thin. Okay, so now I probably remember kids I knew at college who had similar problems and I give the guy a twenty-pound note.

That simple act of reaching out starts a process of reflection that is already subtly altering how I see myself in the world: I would not hand over my hard-earned cash unless I thought that by doing so, I was changing something for the better. Hopefully it helps the person I gave it to. But being generous also helps me: suddenly, I am more aware of how lucky I am to have children who love me and still like to visit me, and to have a good, regular income. I may feel a surge of compassion for people who are homeless or down on their luck. Instead of being so preoccupied with work, I start to notice other people. My focus widens. When I get home, I close the curtains against the rain and recall that I have half a dozen jackets I never wear hanging in the cupboard, so I choose a warm coat, a hat, a scarf and some gloves and put them in a bag; and the next day, I see the same guy and give him the bag of clothes. He immediately puts on the gloves and winds the scarf around his shoulders. Now I feel really good. I did something that made a positive difference. I am probably already seeing the world differently and will choose to work differently and make decisions from a subtly altered perspec-tive. That is spiritual progress.

We tend to think of significant change as something loud, sudden and dramatic – BOOM! – shaking us up like a bottle of lemonade. And that can happen. Even so, important change is often the result of very subtle decisions, small choices and chance encounters that cumulatively alter our understanding over a long period. As I have found, changes usually arrive in small dosages, so that we accept them more easily.

Spiritual Laws are constant and unchanging, even as they change the world around us constantly. We can apply them to any set of circumstances. Thus, there is no such thing as a hopeless case or a dead end. Instead there arises a constant stream of opportunities to see and do things differently. As we apply these laws, increasingly we notice them working. When we believe them, they are exponentially effective. Thus, if we nurture respectful and loving thoughts about ourselves, we discover that Universal wisdom unfolds more easily and joyfully to assist us. The truth of our value and worth in the world becomes increasingly self-evident and powerful, helping us to focus with greater clarity as we listen more closely and refine our understandings. Gradually we accept the joyful discipline of paying careful attention and acting according to our highest beliefs about ourselves.

If humankind is to succeed in the longer term, we must become more aware that the world of opposites we inhabit and that seems so puzzling and unfair – big/small, poor/rich, success/failure, good/bad – hides a greater truth that all states of being co-exist. Through an ongoing process of expanding awareness, first we notice that we are constantly choosing between "opposites"; then we notice that this scheme of choices exists for a purpose: without the Everything we can choose from, we could not experience the Emptiness within which Everything is held. Without hot, there could be no cold; without sorrow, happiness would have no meaning. Unless we can have *some* awareness of lack, success on any level – knowing ourselves to be loved, appreciated and understood, for example – would be very difficult to notice. Our world of opposites exists to allow us to appreciate different states of existence. At the same time, we start to perceive our unity with all shades of being. Thus, our precious individuality masks a reality that at a different level, we are fundamentally the same. Appreciating the usefulness of this scheme, we can consciously deploy the illusion of differences to choose experiences we prefer.

For example, in the midst of feelings of lack, we decide to count our blessings because by doing so, we renew our experience of feeling abundantly blessed. I may give something to someone in need, so that they may feel good about themselves, and so that I may experience that I have it to give; a cycle which helps us all to feel prosperous. In sharing, we disarm unhappiness, just as our hoarding causes great and unnecessary grief.

Illusions of difference, separation and disunity, serve us by allowing us to choose to experience and appreciate different, more connected states and conditions of being. And when we know we are playing this game, we can and often do feel two "opposing" states at once: blessed and sorrowful, loved and excluded, happy and sad. Thus, the final illusion – that we are separate from each other – allows us to experience our unity with all things. In experiencing again our grandness, we use the illusions of this world as they are intended to be used, to experience our choices playing out as we make them, and in hopefully choosing to move towards more loving and peaceful attitudes.

We are lost in the illusions of separateness when we believe they are real and they keep us trapped in a world governed by appearances and material needs; we find the Divine in each other, when we use the illusions to notice our grand unity with all things.

FREE WILL

Because we cannot physically see the energy of our choices moving forward and shaping our future, we learn, and are taught, to take the majority of our beliefs on trust. Yet, even when we live in total ignorance that there are any such things as universal laws or processes, whether we consider that life's outcomes are the result of chance, fate or bad luck has no real effect on the ways in which the physical laws of the universe coalesce around us.

Free will is the belief that, despite what we may feel about our place in the world, we are always free to exercise choices, without fear of retribution, punishment or guilt. The fundamental importance of free will is obscured in the many ways we surrender our power and in the ways that society currently organizes itself, so that many people believe they have no free will whatsoever. We may have a really hard life, and so it is challenging to accept that directly or indirectly, we create or contribute to our circumstances.

I cannot explain exactly how it is that I have

come along the path towards accepting that certain attitudes, beliefs and behaviours are more beneficial than others; perhaps it is a simple matter of navigating from choices that feel less good to those that feel better. Yet I know, mainly through personal experience, that agreeing I have freedom to choose is of paramount importance if I want to make progress towards a happier life. Despite deeply rooted resistance to this notion, I have to admit that even the briefest glimpse of my freedom helps me to handle daily limitations with greater maturity and work with challenges more deliberately to shape my life.

Once we start to accept that the power of our personal free will works at every level – at any level that feels comfortable – immediately our focus shifts to what we can do now to make our lives more meaningful, more joyful and increasingly purposeful. Whatever may have happened in the past is of limited importance. It is what I am deciding and doing now that shapes my life. As with anything, practice makes perfect.

In exercising our spiritual muscles, there is no better place to witness results than with ourselves. Each massive undertaking, even the grandest ambition, begins with a small decision, a tiny step, a fresh resolve. And once we start to flex the power of our free will as we align it with our conscious choices, we naturally begin from the assumption that every choice, big or small, makes a difference. Our choices all impact each other.

At a higher level, free will invites us to accept that life blesses us with amazing opportunities. Whatever choices we make, no higher power is going to come along and disapprove, or punish us for making "wrong" choices. Instead, each decision we make, each road we choose, becomes our opportunity to restate and reconsider, "How do I like to feel? What do I wish to offer in this situation? What impact is my behaviour having now?"

I may decide to commit to a relationship. Having decided, I encounter other avenues and responsibilities: of mutual respect, nurture and faithfulness. I may then choose to have children, which brings further choices and added responsibilities of caring, nurture, love and affection. In order to honour the choices I have made, I am helped when I recall that these decisions were originally in my power and my choice to make and I must have made them for a reason, probably because I believed they would make me happy. I love having a responsibility to act in ways that make me happy.

None of us consciously chooses to act in ways that make us miserable. Yet harbouring beliefs that we are worthless, friendless, alone or penniless neither sustains us nor makes our lives comfortable: the power inherent in creative freedom has the result that, whatever we believe about ourselves, we cannot help but see around us the evidence of these truths. Our beliefs give added strength to what we observe. So if we believe our circumstances are pitiable, that is what we see, and so the cycle continues. We may spend years making poor, sorry or harmful choices. Eventually we notice, in glimmers of light, that when we make happier, liberating choices, everyone benefits. I suppose you might call this process part of growing up or getting wiser. Accepting our free will in these situations is ultimately very liberating.

It makes not the slightest difference how small or grand an idea may be. It matters that we have an idea, lots of ideas, that we plant them in the soil of our determination and allow them space and encouragement to grow. Each tree begins as a hope of the mother tree. Each leaf unfolds boldly in springtime. So it is with our hopes, our choices and our decisions.

CAUSE AND EFFECT

Cause and effect are simple enough concepts to grasp, reminding us that all of our choices have consequences. We are all choosing all the time; and the ways in which our choices mix and mingle produce results which are often complex and unseen. Nevertheless, our decisions are respected – because we have free will – so it serves us to think the best of ourselves and to do the best we can, with the highest and most sincere motivation we can muster. It sounds easy and obvious and at a more practical level, it is: I go to the store for a litre of milk, I have to pay for it; I steal it, I get caught; I get caught, the police may let me off with a warning or they may throw the book at me…

Whatever way we choose to go, we get to live with the consequences. So, we help ourselves to make life easier when we choose to act in ways that are loving, thoughtful, caring, decisive, patient, hard-working, loyal, forgiving… And it is helpful to foster and encourage beliefs that Life supports us, people are kind, the world is a peaceful place and that every plan we have and nurture will come to fruition in the best way possible.

If cause and effect work at a practical level, they probably work at lots of different emotional, mental and spiritual levels too. I happen to believe this is true, because when I am kind and forgiving, increasingly I notice that the world is easier to live in; when I am thoughtful and hard-working, I reap dividends; and when I believe that Life helps me with all my decisions, I feel inspired and loved in everything. I simply gather up enjoyable qualities and deploy them as consciously as I can. As I do, opportunities flower around me, gradually quieting the voices of incredulity and hardship.

It is like learning to ski. Though I will never feel the exhilaration of catching a lift to the top of the mountainside, of flying downhill, soaring and dipping, even so I can apply a similar analogy to the ways in which our successes come about. If I am on the slide, that will tend to bring about circumstances that justify my feelings. When I feel exhilarated, filled with excited energy, the consequences are likely to be exciting and my excited energy attracts to me more of the same. This is how cause and effect play, hand in hand with all the other laws, including free will and the law of attraction. If we will relax and allow it to do so, the whole of life continually conspires in our favour, helping at every stage and stopping post.

THE LAW OF ATTRACTION

No matter how earnestly my mind takes up its disputatious cudgels, the evidence of my life continually offers proof that respecting How Life Works brings dividends and insights which grow clearer and more convincing with use. That these precepts may be hard to explain rationally or logically seems rather beside the point: I only care that by applying them, I can see how they work, which encourages me to live more effectively. Whether I want to or not, I see all the ways in which refusing to listen to guidance hurts me – and others – while honouring these principles enhances my life.

The law of magnetism reminds us that our internal power source continually draws towards us the circumstances in our lives. Around our bodies, which are simply the vehicles we need in order to express the workings of our spirits on planet Earth, our souls dance continually, the magic of their magnetic, pulsing energy pulling inexorably, and attracting a variety of situations and outcomes and keeping away others which are set on a different frequency. Our habitual frequency, whether it is set to high or is dipping a bit low, brings into our lives largely what we expect it to.

We are attractive to someone when we notice them, they notice us and we click. They speak to our interests, they answer some excitement in us and there is an indefinable buzz. We pull towards them and search out life events and preferences we share, consciously and unconsciously bringing ourselves closer together. When we fall in love, we see the best of everything in the other person. (We say, rather dismissively, that love is blind. This is surprisingly true. True love accepts all. Real love is remarkably pure and forgiving, precisely because it does not distinguish, but loves in all conditions.)

Magnetism and attraction are constantly at work, pulling together forces that are mutually attractive and repelling those that are not. Thus, our normal emotional frequency pulls towards us all the people and events we "expect" and keeps away all those other things we do not expect, whether "good" or "bad". We may fall out of love. Small irritations start to grate and annoy and we become less tolerant of mistakes and misunderstandings. We begin to repel and naturally move apart, perhaps because our frequency is falling, while that of the other person remains constant. Or it may be that we are growing into a different frequency that another person doesn't "get".

Our usual "broadband" frequency, though set at some point which we would regard as "normal", is capable of constant change; and interestingly, it can vary, depending on which role we are in at any time. We may be a superbly confident business person, able to attract all the resources we need to easily secure fantastic outcomes, while, at home, we struggle with our personal relationships and find it hard to maintain a conversation. Distinctions like these are not usually so marked, but if this sounds familiar, we might pause to consider why we allow such a disparity to continue.

We can consciously think about, and attract, great ideas, wonderful outcomes, supportive friends and superb opportunities to support us, whatever we are doing. The Universe helps us to recognize when we are achieving these, because when we feel good, we achieve more positive results. We feel better, more alive and purposeful when we maintain ourselves with large doses of self-belief and self-encouragement. Learning to love ourselves unconditionally is an immensely powerful way in which we can raise our magnetic frequency to attract more beneficial outcomes.

There is no judgement in this process, no opinion offered as to whether a course of action or belief system is "better" or "worse". We only have to decide which outcomes we prefer, which will usually – but not always – be those which make us feel better. It is interesting to reflect how many of us tolerate a level of suffering, discomfort or deprivation, in the mistaken belief that these are inevitable. It can be hard, when we feel deprived and unhappy, to notice that anything else is possible. It can be very challenging to step away from our usual sluggish frequencies and decide, "You know, I really would like to feel better than this!"

Even though we may dream of feeling happier, more comfortable and more confident, we may lack the self-belief that we can make it so; we can't believe that our mere choices, such small, fragile things, can have life-changing impact.

We can and they do: the Universe takes every opportunity to remind us of our power and to help and guide us along paths that we will find most rewarding. Becoming aware of how we would prefer to feel and how we can shift our habitual frequencies higher through respecting what we enjoy, we start a process that carries us towards a more comfortable future.

THE LAW OF REFLECTION

As we accept and work with spiritual wisdom, we may see life unfolding for us in many ways as we expect it to. Instead of cluttering our lives up with incessant mental chatter, for example, we wait silently and learn to live deeply in the Now. Knowing that our thoughts and beliefs are creative, as profound peace takes over our lives, we notice that people, choices and circumstances arrive beside us, brought towards us by what we expect.

Life works this way. Our beliefs are reflected in what we experience. If we believe in poverty and striving, we will be poor and strive. If we are paralyzed with fear at the prospect of undertaking a new task, people attracted to us, whether personally or professionally, will mirror our level of fear or (lack of) self-belief and will inevitably have their own issues that naturally reinforce our own beliefs. If we had not been at that level, we would not have attracted them to us. If we then blame them, perhaps for not being supportive or for not doing what we expect of them, we are essentially blaming them for being attracted to us, when so often, it is we who have brought our circumstances into our lives, with our unconscious beliefs.

To become free from this, it helps to accept that the Universe is working around us all the time, with all the circumstances and material we are offering up, to procure the best possible outcome it can for us. We can work with Life or we can fight it. We can resist, or we can harness the processes of attraction, reflection, and cause and effect to work for us while we do our best, whatever happens. Living calmly and happily in the Now and giving out lovingly in the midst of the daily round, offers us our best opportunities because we are beautiful and deserve to be happy.

CREATIVE CHOICES

So, do we have our paintbrushes ready? We've got our easel propped up there, against that wall, and a palette of colours ready to daub on the canvas… What are we going to paint? How we work the canvas is entirely up to us. It feels daunting, almost like leaping off a cliff, when we decide to commit that first line, risk a smudge of red or blue, sketching first outlines of a ghost of an idea so tentatively. When we start out, that is what we do, drawing careful, light lines, which gradually firm up as our decisions are made.

Why do we sometimes feel as if success and happiness happen to other people? While all around us, others prosper and laugh, we scrimp and save, we are calculating and careful, and yet there is never quite enough. Our time is divided uneasily among six or eight different concerns, while our own projects sit neglected, gathering dust. Our energy is expended on several daily preoccupations that see us untidily through the day. Our money is spent on household needs, on children's clothes, on bills and insurance. What about us?

Undoubtedly, my tendency to put things off, to wait and see, to calculate or weigh up endless possibilities and try to anticipate everything that might go wrong, makes it that bit harder for solutions and success to flow towards me. But I suspect that other factors are at play.

How many of us accept wholeheartedly that we deserve to be happy or successful? How many of us actively welcome hope and joy into our lives? Readers of my earlier book may remember what I wrote there, about recognizing success and accepting it for ourselves. Such a fundamental part of creativity can be looked at again. I hope you will bear with me as I reconsider what it means to recognize and welcome success into our lives.

It is a fundamental rule that unless we see our success, we cannot be successful. "To BE it, SEE it", or if you prefer, "to SEE it, BE it." Unless we recognize that we are happy, wise and free, we cannot be happy, wise or free. Since we are constantly attracting to ourselves That Which We Are or that which we see ourselves as, from all the options available, we may prefer to recognize that, "I *am* successful, I am pleased, I am kind, I am free, I am filled with excitement, I am powerful, I am happy. I am a maker of miracles. My life is a miracle..." All these statements – which gradually morph into certainty – work to produce results that prove us right.

You may notice that as soon as we say, "I am great fun to be around and I have lots of friends" or, "I am such a waste of space and nobody loves me" or even, "you are cruel and thoughtless," our sub-conscious mind automatically goes on the lookout, finding evidence that agrees with us. Whatever the nature of our thoughts, the Universe is obliging: *it always agrees wholeheartedly and matches exactly our own beliefs.* As attraction works, once we notice that we are (in fact) happy, we jump-start a process of attracting to ourselves more of that quality, which vindicates our belief and creates more happiness.

"To those that have, shall be given and from those that have not, shall be taken away." (1) For many years, that saying puzzled me, as it seemed unfair and obscure. Then one day I was standing doing a fairly mundane task in the kitchen and I finally under-stood how important it is, to see in and around me all those qualities and assets I desire to experience as part of my life. Unless I notice them within and around me – unless I know they are part of my expe-rience – how can I hope to attract them?

I may say, "I Am Successful", daring the Universe to disagree with me. Automatically my thoughts begin to cast around, observing in the ten thousand small steps I have already taken to get here, how much

I have achieved. In noticing how far I have already travelled from despair to happiness and from failure to success, accepting that I am successful then becomes so much more obvious, and my continued denials sound hollow even to me. In that moment, while peeling vegetables in the kitchen, I understood that any small acceptance of my achievements opens the gates for more of the same to surround me.

Our noticing, appreciating or loving *any* quality or aspect brings more of that same quality to us, whether that is poverty, loneliness and difficulty; or peace, acceptance, love and happiness. It sounds easy when I write it all down and nod my head. It sounds obvious, but how many of us turn away our blessings a hundred times a day without realizing?

I woke one morning and my first thought was, "I would love a hot drink." Exactly on cue my husband walked into the bedroom with a delicious, steaming cup of chicory. Did I smile, reach up and gratefully accept the proffered drink? No, I absent-mindedly placed the mug on the bedside table. While its contents were good and hot and I would have relished the heat, did I drink gratefully? No, I left my cup to cool to an unattractive sludge and later swallowed it with a distinct lack of enthusiasm.

Automatically, I turned away my blessing. From long habit, I have dismissed my joys – the things I love – as being of little importance, or, at any rate, much less important than anything else that I "have to" make time for. As I continually put off doing what I want to do, opportunities and activities that I would enjoy hover at the periphery, waiting patiently for the day when I will turn to them gladly. Thankfully, that morning I suddenly noticed what I had done, was able to write about it in my journal and laugh about it. At last, I glimpsed some of my own responsibility for pushing away my good fortune.

A habit of discounting or ignoring whatever I would most like to do has crept up over the years and is liable to infect every choice I would make about my family, my career and my loves. I have to be careful that Eddie and Seline don't take me too seriously when I say that I am "happy enough staying here" as they go off by themselves on some weekend adventure. Though I do relish being alone and they certainly need time together without me, I do enjoy being with them. We deserve to do family stuff together. I would hate them to assume that I never expect to be invited.

Doing what I want to do has value for its own sake. Knowing this, I can begin to reawaken my honest preferences and in that way, gently dismantle an old tendency to appear indifferent or put a brave face on some weak compromise. Undoing old habits takes patience and, for some of us, lots of time, since habits cling like glue, even when they sit on us uncomfortably. I have always been impatient to see results now, immediately. I have a similar impatience when it comes to ancient habits: I want them all to evaporate quickly but they lie around, waiting to trip me up when I act thoughtlessly.

I have found it so hard to express my preferences clearly and then wait peacefully with them, resisting the urge to apologize or change my mind, or go the other way and become insistent and angry. Once we have chosen what we want, if we can then allow that to manifest by a process of expectant waiting – genuinely doing nothing – that process is far more likely to produce a happy outcome than worrying and over-thinking.

When I refuse a lovely drink ("not now"), I am resisting my own happiness, which I do in countless ways. We all do, to a greater or lesser degree. Perhaps because we are in a hurry or in the middle of some other task which we think needs to be finished before we can let our hair down, we put off doing what would make us happiest right now. I used to postpone my pleasures forever.

I am continually challenged by a strong underlying resistance to my new choices which shows up as the habit of being overly obliging and in finding excellent, well-argued reasons not to do what I would like to do. Both tendencies are so ingrained that it has taken me years to notice their detrimental effects. What a minefield it can be, picking our way past these rocks to the smoother path of our true enjoyment.

Resistance to change hides buried deep in our past, in fears we formed and in coping habits we used to cover our fears, which crystallized for reasons we have now forgotten. But reactive habits based in fear cannot hide forever, because sooner or later we rediscover the peace and strength that comes from respecting our joy. These days I am very aware of those flashes of unconscious resistance so its days are numbered.

RESISTANCE IS FUTILE

I dreamed of a peaceful ocean which I could see flowing all around me, moving slowly on its way, unstoppable. I was standing shakily at the shoreline, watching the surging blue tide advance steadily towards me. Trying to move out of its way by clambering up the sand, I found that although the beach was cleaner and brighter up here, it made no difference as far as the ocean was concerned: its solid weight continued advancing, waiting for me to accept that it was coming and that escape was impossible. I knew that I had no choice but to join the ocean and float away with it wherever it went.

The ocean of our desires is strong, just as the pull of the tide is irresistible. I would be joining it eventually, so I might as well make the choice to go with the flow and enjoy letting the water carry me peacefully towards fulfilment – where else would Life bring me?

On another occasion I had been asking fretfully, "If the River of Life is inevitable, why is it so uncomfortable?" and a man came and showed me that because I was standing up to my neck in the River, I was creating resistance, hindering the movement of my desires in any peaceful way. It is far easier and more relaxing if, as he showed me, I can float and let the River carry me.

We may push and pull, we may run away and hide, though eventually we must rest. Even the most determined of us has to stop, eventually. We may maim our outer world as well as the inner space of our desires, yet our wishes and dreams will always find a way to resurface in peaceful moments while daydreaming and sleeping. No matter how far we retreat within our towers of concrete and steel, we are part of nature and intimately connected with every natural process. We may cut the grass but it grows back. If the gardeners stopped tending the hedges and edges, thousands of trees would root in the cracks beside the roads all over the city and a curtain of green would quickly overtake all our futile efforts at control, unimpeded by herbicides, lawn mowers or tarmac. That is Life. Life will not be controlled, channelled or cut off for long. Eventually we will understand that nothing can get in the way of Life.

In the same way, miracles are all around us. That we do not see them suggests only that we are not in the habit of noticing them and do not expect to find them near us any time soon. You may read of an Indian holy man and go on a pilgrimage to receive his blessing. But that is not necessary. You may fly hundreds of miles to rediscover your sense of purpose or to locate the meaning of life. But that is a long way to go. You may spend years seeking to discover wisdom, listening to learned teachers and absorbing the teaching of centuries, while right at your side a small miracle is waiting, hoping to be noticed. Miracles are everywhere, because we are miracles.

Understanding that we are part of the miracle and that miracles are inseparable from us, turns our lives around. When we sit still, when we let go, we witness miracles playing around us all the time. Depending on what we ask for, small chances or major break-throughs can become as commonplace as doing the shopping or collecting the dry cleaning, all because we give up the need for control. We stop trying to apply our thoughts to everything and release our beliefs about what we think we understand.

Trying to know everything is a futile chase, pro-ducing an atmosphere where perversely, explana-tions flee and miracles wilt in the heat of our scrutiny. How barren our hopes and dreams would be, if everything in them could be understood by us. I love the secretive. I adore mystery and I try to cultivate a respectful silence around those things which are simply too multi-layered to get my head round. Some things, I am pleased to know, are not meant to be understood. Reaching the final edge of understanding would be like asking, "What is the biggest number?" and discovering the answer. Endings imply that the infinite is quantifiable.

The creative power we call Life, Source, or Love cannot be controlled, counted, or even fully understood. That is not our part in the exercise, nor, I believe, why we are here. We are always part of Life, though we cannot really control what Life Is. If we want to learn a bit more, we can stop searching so frantically. Searching for miracles, they flee. If we wait quietly in welcome and invitation, they draw nearer to us gladly.

With my intellect, I understand why resistance is pointless. Physical and mental resisting take up lots of energy. Worrying, thinking too hard, planning everything exactly or trying to figure out every permutation are time-consuming. And outcomes are not changed as much as we expect by the effort we invest with our fighting attitude. The question we can ask ourselves is, "Do we want a wonderful life or a life filled with pain?"

When we aim to make changes for the better, when we are hoping to walk forward more confidently and cheerfully, sometimes we find it hard to understand why, then, we stumble and fall, why we watch our plans unravel as difficulties crowd round and pester us. If we are tired or careless, we can start to believe that our efforts for change are pointless.

Say, for example, that I know I am being a bad-tempered wife who takes her husband for granted. I'm angry because I'm exhausted and it is too long since I did anything remotely enjoyable: been there, done that. One day I decide I have to start behaving better, and I do, for a while. For a few days or weeks, I am gentler with myself, I make a point of relaxing more and I find lots of calming happiness within me which comes to the surface after years of neglect. I begin to truly believe that actually, I *am* truly a wonderful person and that I *can* stay peaceful, whatever pressures come my way. I become more careful, kind and considerate. Gentle words greet my husband on his return home; and I enjoy cooking tasty, restoring meals, I really, honestly do. Thus, life improves for us. My vibrations are climbing nicely, when all of a sudden, I find myself in the middle of a huge domestic row. How did that happen and why, when I was sincerely working to change? How can life be so unkind that way?

Often, lapses are down to unfamiliarity with the new, the ease of falling back into old habits and an underlying resistance to change. If you are sitting forward nodding, I suggest that you read or reread the sections about resistance in my earlier book, *Happiness Matters*. There, I give many examples which show how easily things can go wrong when we are working for positive change, tempting us to give up our hopes for renewal as a bad idea. Accidents and reversals happen because our older mind habits perceive *all* change as threatening, and neither recognize nor accept that any change in our attitude is positive or beneficial.

Consciously, we know that good changes make us feel happier, more contented, more relaxed and fulfilled. We have more energy and smile more. Even so, our layers of deeper mind do not, and probably cannot, distinguish between behaviour that might be unhelpful – old, negative habits – and new, happier patterns we are hoping to take on board. Our deeper minds only prefer that we should always stay the same, not rock the boat. Life is less threatening that way. Old and familiar is better than new and challenging, any day. Resistance – things "going wrong" when we least expect them to – is simply good old-fashioned Fear of Change; fear which does not distinguish between "good" or "bad" changes.

Some recent examples show how deeply entrenched resistance can be:

~ I am singing a happy tune around the house, then immediately fall and bang my hip. (Fear replies, "No, you are not really happy after all.")

~ When someone asks me how I am, I reply, "Fine, thank you!" and then practically fall on top of them. (Fear is saying, "Actually, you are not fine.")

~ There is a film I would really love to go and see at the cinema, but I forget to make concrete plans. When my husband reminds me he has a meeting the same evening, I let him go without mentioning my own plans. (Resistance is saying, "Your plans are less important than other people's," or "You do not deserve/need/really want to go out.")

~ The printer jams, the scanner needs replacing, the computer gets a virus, its hard-drive packs in… (Resistance is suggesting I give up trying to do what I would usually enjoy.)

~ At the swimming pool, I am happily saying to myself, "From now on, I fully intend to be preoccupied with happy thoughts – it's about time!" Then I slip on a top step as I'm getting into the water and twist my foot awkwardly so that for weeks afterwards I can hardly walk. The pain is excruciating and lasts for two full months. (Resistance is saying, "No! Have something unpleasant to preoccupy you, like you usually do.")

Are we strong enough to accept the obstacles that land in our path and say about them, "Well, you aren't going to stop me feeling good, I am going to stay with my refreshing intentions, no matter what you throw at me."?

Instead of asking, "Why does this always happen to me?" or "Why does my life always have to be so difficult?" perhaps a better question is, "What am I frightened of?" As a new writer, my existence was festooned with stop-start situations through which part of me doggedly insisted on keeping going. Despite endless setbacks, I could see over a period of years that forward momentum was steady, though in tiny steps. At times, underlying resistance tested my patience – and the love of my family – to the limit. Despite small but definite signs of progress, some part of me was still frightened of going forward with my plans and of thinking that I could actually claim any new exciting adventures for myself – "The higher you climb, the harder you fall!"

For years, I have been afraid of success, fearing that sharp criticism would follow in its wake. With every sinew in my body tuned to hear the voices of criticism rather than encouragement, none was louder than my own. So I have tended to sabotage my work first, before someone else might criticize it and, as I then saw it, effectively end my progress and hopes of eventual success. I have feared public humiliation, which has tended to go in the same basket as personal annihilation. Since this particular fear goes back decades, it is deeply rooted and, being very familiar, it is surprisingly good at passing unnoticed.

When I forget to reassure myself, my subconscious, looking for ways to protect me, helps with some handy sabotage now and then. As deadlines and new decisions approach and even as I assert my freedom and happiness in making choices which fill me with joy, or which bring financial rewards and recognition, I dither, or there is a reaction: I fall and bang my head, I break things and have to spend ages gluing them together; I delay, while the clock ticks and my appointment draws nearer. It makes a twisted kind of sense, but it is a strange knot which has taken years to unravel and learn to deal with.

We can make a useful parallel with a child who, growing older, ventures daily beyond his usual boundaries. For a while he is happy with new discoveries and he feels free. Then, just as mother ponders how terribly grown up he is for his age, he feels a bit of fear and comes running back to mummy's side, where he feels safe again, before venturing out once more on his own and going a little further ahead into the big wide world.

Our minds are like that too. They tend to find any change in our attitudes threatening, until gradually assimilated and accepted as part of our "normal" behaviour. So instead of ranting and raving at a computer – I don't want that to be my normal behaviour! – I can reassure myself, "This is fear of success. Now that I am choosing peace and meaningful work for myself there is nothing to fear and everything to gain. Every situation is safe and I am protected; there is nothing to fear and much to rejoice in. All works out well for me." If you prefer humour, smile and say, "Well, I don't care what you believe, I *am* happy, I *am successful.* And if this computer is kaput, then I'll go and get another one!"

To give another example, I may be aiming to improve my health, recognizing my physical strengths and saying, "I am healthy and happy." All goes well for a few days and weeks. I have more energy as increasingly I recognize around me all the convincing evidence that I am indeed healthy and strong. Then suddenly a head cold pops up out of nowhere and my body aches. Or my back hurts and my throat feels raw.

Such minor niggles are part of my body's attempts to protect me by lowering my vibration so that I get back to what the body recognizes as my more usual frequency. My body is trying to help, so getting cross will make annoying niggles worse. Instead, I try to laugh them off or sing cheerful songs at the top of my voice. Remembering that my mind is powerful and controls my body, I focus with clarity and determination on my intention to remain happy and, indeed, to continue to grow towards ever greater fulfilment. Reassurance, a laugh and a little time to rest – and to notice what is happening – are often enough to ease the aches and pains. Persisting with hopes for change is never a waste. Every gram of optimism helps to make the shift.

So if and when you find yourself sitting in a puddle of tears wailing, "Why, oh, why is this happening? Why me?" it might help console you to ponder what situation has recently changed that your mind finds threatening. What unfamiliar territory have you moved into? Have you posted off a job application, or are you thinking of putting your home on the market? Are you in a new romance and unsure where it might take you?

So long as you know that you are pleased with your new choices, keep intending them. Keep seeing yourself moving into lighter happier places, while understanding that annoying disasters that crop up are fairly typical backlash, like a speedboat cutting through water and raising a drenching spray. How strong a reversal is, depends on how deep a fear goes. Deep-rooted fears may be taking a long time to surface, unhook themselves and leave. Meantime, lots of reassurance, gentleness and personal kindness are more helpful than anger or guilt. You might wish to send up a prayer or ask for help to identify what particular fear your body is reacting to and how you may best calm it. Meantime, keep using positive actions and words to lift yourself up. ("Well done! This is hard, but I'm doing really well.")

Since I understand that there is never a time when I am not asking and choosing, I can ask more easily now. I ask for help with this plan or that problem. A much more personal challenge for me has been to accept that my choices are worthwhile and to allow myself to embrace them fully now and for always. So, in answer to that particular challenge, I can assert, "I always deserve to be happy and to enjoy myself. I am always worthy to have fun. When I am happy, everyone benefits. My choices are worthy. In my choices are Life's expression and service."

If there is a backlash, it becomes ever clearer to me that there has never been a better time to dismantle and disarm a scrap more of my underlying resistance with yet more patient gentleness.

> I dreamed of a cartoon figure, like an Asterix centurion, a woman with a shock of white hair which was clamped carelessly under an unfastened helmet. Perhaps she was first employed as a bodyguard, many years ago. She is holding a bayonet at a careless slant and the effort is clearly telling. Her ancient frame, always diminutive, is now bent over and she is long overdue to retire, very obviously ineffective.
>
> Message – your aged fears are long overdue to retire. They are comical and no longer needed. Nor are they effective in holding you back from progress in your life. You can safely ask them to leave now. You do not need their protection – you have nothing to fear.

PROBABLE OUTCOMES

Imagine that you have arrived at a Y junction and there are two possible routes you can choose to travel. One is more favourable than the other. Compare, "You will meet the love of your life this year" and "Your resolve will be greatly tested in the next twelve months." Do you:

(a)Focus on the less desirable possibility and try to psyche yourself up for it?

(b)Focus on the more desirable outcome, even if you feel it is unlikely?

(c)Ignore both predictions and get on with your life?

(d)Feel confused and give up altogether?

Out of interest, I asked my husband what he would do. He replied immediately that he would focus on the poorer outcome and try to prepare for the worst. On my bad days, I freely admit, I am tempted to give up altogether and never leave bed again.

What got me energised was remembering the more helpful option, which is to (b) focus on the outcome which feels most desirable. If that doesn't work, at least I can (c) ignore both predictions and get on with my life the best I can.

If taking control of our lives means anything, it means remembering the power we hold within us to choose all the time. Everything we think, say and do is making our future. Every one of our intentions and actions is the result of our focus on *something*. As we live in an attraction-based universe, we cannot help attracting things to us: our thinking about them makes them ever more likely to occur in our experience.

So rather than seeing ourselves as helpless and lost, a butterfly buffeted by unpredictable circumstances beyond our control, it is more cheerful if we conjure up and intend a better outcome – as wonderful as we wish – and focus on that. We feel better and the more cheerful hope is increasingly likely to come true. If we gently look beyond the more difficult alternatives, they tend to either evaporate or wither and die from lack of attention. Even if our desired results take a while to arrive – say, two to three years instead of the one year given in this example – in all that time we will have been happier. Happiness for its own sake is a brilliant result, whatever else we might be hoping for.

We probably find it difficult to maintain a resolutely optimistic mind. Our intentions and certainties tend to waver as time passes; and as we notice people around us caught up with their difficulties, we remember our own problems. That may be one reason why our desires take a while to show up: while positive intentions and courage will tend to speed up good outcomes, thoughtless pessimism hinders them; and if we keep changing our minds all the time, it is little wonder that Life becomes confused.

I have been in the habit of consulting psychics and mediums for answers to my questions. When will things get easier? Is there a reason for all this difficulty? Can you explain why it has to be like this? And on and on... My questions become more anguished as the months pass. Meanwhile, all this time, another part of me *knows* I am very lucky. I receive constant reassurances in dreams, happy coincidences, even dream messages in numbers. Yet, even knowing that help is all around me, I have tended to ferret out the one negative comment in a sea of praise. I have been so like that person who organizes a conference and instead of congratulating myself for having it all run smoothly, I give myself a hard time because I forgot to order flowers for the top table.

Whatever we are doing, we cannot help bringing our focus and energy to this path, that preference, this or that attitude or belief. And in so doing, we naturally bring our choices closer towards us. We can kick our happier ambitions into the long grass by being inattentive, careless, negative or habitually grumpy. Some parts of our lives can be predicted quite far into the future. Other parts, the complexions of our choices…? Well, these are our responsibility. Our powerful focus affects every possible outcome. That is why predictions are vague: they may not happen and, despite all the predictions, we can choose otherwise.

At every hand and turn, we navigate our own lives. And so, if you are ever faced with a choice of what to think or what to believe, you may prefer to aim for that choice which lifts you up, the path that fills you with hope and energy. The secret of success in any enterprise is to decide what we prefer and stick with it. If we can make up our minds for cheerfulness, we are giving ourselves the best present we can.

WHAT ARE WE WAITING FOR?

How often have we said or thought, "I will spring-clean my house when…", "I'll paint a picture after I have…" or, "I'll book a holiday when I've finished doing…" We frustrated, unfulfilled people have a bad habit. We decide we will do (what makes us happy when we have finished doing) what we ought to do first. We postpone our bliss, expecting it to wait for us indefinitely, as we shelve it out of sight or add it as an afterthought at the bottom of our list of things to do *some day*, once we have grown up, married, once we have raised the children and finished ironing shirts.

Meanwhile, going about our everyday lives, we plot and dig, we push and shove.

Why do we press on regardless of our health, of our need to eat, rest and play? We don't consider actually doing now what we enjoy, because we are too busy worrying about the security of our jobs, our homes, our possessions and our lives. Every year brings gloomy news of financial or economic crisis which we take so seriously, even though we know that such attitudes make us feel heavy. We tend to become increasingly frantic when we are looking for something that we cannot find.

Will we ever be finished with that list of things that need doing? Are we ready, now? Or do you need permission to go fetch your bliss? Whenever we take our courage in both hands and go right ahead and do first what we most long to do, there we find joy, where it has been waiting for us all along. If you still need someone to give you the go-ahead, I bless you for this. I do.

If something is so important to us that, even contemplating it, we want to sing and dance and think in colour and burst with pride…why do we allow it to languish dusty and unloved on the bottom shelf of our ambition? Give it love. Feed it. In other words – do it NOW. Do it first! Do it immediately. Do not wait around to see what happens. Do not wait to win the lottery. Do not ask for my opinion. Stop waiting for the postman or for your husband or wife to come home, for the phone to ring. Stop hanging around, waiting for your mother to come – and go again – so that you can "get on". Get on with what? Housework? Is *that* why we have breath and life? Unless we are cooks or homemakers, unless that is our heart's desire, we can afford to cut ourselves some slack.

Be happy first. Give that first fresh burst of energy in your day to whoever or whatever you love the most. Every small moment of joy is precious and irreplaceable and in every moment, we can decide to be happy. If we love to write, let's write first. If it is painting, let's get our paints and brushes out of their boxes. If it is laughing and singing, let's do some of that while our energy is light and fresh and we are most open to guidance.

Whenever we have the courage to leave aside for a moment that list of "things we have to do" and trust our first impulse, we often receive some form of confirmation or validation that lifts and carries us further in a good direction: we feel more relaxed; we laugh for the first time in months; the weight seems to shift from our shoulders and chest; our days feel easier and we sleep better at night; other people are suddenly more agreeable; the weather improves. When we have decided to be happy (and yes, we can simply decide, one day, that this is what we will be!) Life can and does challenge us and throws all kinds of dramas at our feet in an attempt to derail our optimism. But, since we have decided, we can remain unruffled and calm. Eventually the dramas get sorted out, the kinks in the cloth of our life are smoothed away.

When we give our priorities another look and decide that, for a change, we are going to give our passions some space to breathe, the satisfaction of our enthusiasm calms us. Personal fulfilment makes us peaceful individuals so that we curb our excesses. These are wonderful reasons to make room for everything we prefer.

Silence that flows from a genuine desire to be still is revitalizing and valuable. A contemplative attitude can be helpful – even essential – to help us find our way and to clarify our next steps. However, as an obedient answer to our expectations and the needs of others, constantly silencing our desires – dismissing what makes us feel alive – spells a slow, suffocating death of talent, joy and opportunity. That almost happened to me. I almost never wrote my first book and might still be sitting in that armchair under the window, doing nothing much except perhaps reading about the lives of other people. Please, have the courage to enjoy your talents and watch as your life becomes a continuous miracle.

VERTICAL TIME

I was walking peacefully alongside a row of shops near my home. There are a couple of charity shops there, and that morning I decided quite firmly to visit the second. As soon as I decided, my brain started arguing, "*Why not the other one? What's wrong with the other shop?*" The ego likes an argument and it would be the same argument whichever shop I chose. Ignoring the head noise, I stayed with my preference. At the cash desk, where I was waiting to hand in some books and oddments, stood a very dear friend whom I meet rarely and who looked up with a broad grin when I called her name. We had an animated chat and exchanged several hugs before going on our way, cheered and uplifted by our chance encounter.

As I stood outside the shop ready to continue with my day, I was very struck by the awareness that in every second, all my choices have consequences, some of which I can't predict: whether to phone or write to someone, whether to go here or there, whether to be peaceful or unhappy. Who knows what effect my decisions will have? There came the thought that time is like a vertical line that connects us to heaven, a line of ideas and outcomes that moves with us vertically, as well as on the horizontal plane – the long and winding road we are familiar with. In every moment, our path unfolds as we move. In each moment as we choose, our thoughts reach ahead of us, if you like, making this or that path or outcome more or less likely. I might not have gone into that shop. I might have walked around the corner, crossed the road or turned around and walked back. I met my friend and we shared such uplifting moments, which I took as validation that I had listened to my preferences and was on the right track.

When we consider the possibility that vertical time is mapping our future with each second, it becomes easier to understand why *A Course In Miracles* (2) reminds us that there is no such thing as an idle thought. Given the immense power that moves our thoughts, there cannot be. Our thoughts make our choices; and our choices make our future as we travel through each day. Considering how many trillions of choices interact to produce outcomes makes me dizzy, though seeing ourselves at the front of our own creative edge is ultimately liberating.

Playing with the possibility of vertical time, I can see how free I am to let go of the past and stop worrying about the future. If my time is a line up to heaven, a small space of choice in the second in which I am standing, then the past is well and truly finished and the future becomes a flexible quantity which I can fill with positive thoughts, as well as uplifting ideas and intentions. All at once, I can see that there is nothing to dread in the future, since I am making it happen as I go along. Even if I am dreading something – going to work, breaking up with my partner, the loss of my home – if the future is re-created one second at a time, I can pump in good feelings, new ideas and energy, with a few prayers for strength and help with the decisions I face.

Vertical time is both reassuring – I am always connected to heaven by my time line – and empowering – nothing truly exists except Now. The past, with all its problems and misunderstandings, is more easily released and so we can unburden ourselves. Every second is filled with the freedom to move this way or that, to explore one possibility or countless others.

> This morning I had a waking dream I fell into, somehow, although I was awake.
>
> I am swimming in beautifully cool and warm alternating currents, then get out and get dressed and start walking. I notice that when I put one foot deliberately in front of the other to climb up the sand to the top

of the beach, the ground, which starts out sandy and shifting, becomes firmer with each step, more certain. Stepping stones rise through the sand to support my feet and make a path before and behind me. The way forms ahead of me, taking me easily up the beach and onto a path which ends in a loop. I could walk round the loop and back down the slope, back to the sea; or I can notice that the path now radiates out in many different directions, depending on where I choose to walk. Clear paths, all of them, uncluttered and smooth.

I want to collect good pebbles to make something, perhaps a road, so I find myself stooping and picking up what I think are sweets, but actually are only the wrappers that someone else has thrown down. I am distracted by the bright colours of the plastic wrappers.

Message: with the certainty of your inner belief, you make your path as you go. You can have a smooth walk up to where you would like to be, but you must keep your head up, keep your focus long and not obsess about details which will hold you back and distract you. Keep moving up the hill and the answers will come, as you go forward.

MAKING SPACE FOR MIRACLES

The joy of life is best seen in its new beginnings; and we are always in a place where we can start again. Small changes in shape and expectation that we choose are not usually greeted with a chorus of disapproval. Thus we learn that we can take bigger steps with ever greater hope, daring to believe that our decisions can lighten our lives. There are strategies we can deploy to help us move ahead with confidence and clarity. If your life and your mind are filled with so much stuff that you have no idea where to begin, perhaps these pointers will help you make more space for miracles.

Overlook Difficulties

I have found that life is refreshing when I learn to overlook difficulties and stay focussed on what better outcomes I prefer. The more I bring my focus down to what's "wrong" with my life, the more real these distracting issues become. My world suddenly grows several shades darker and heavier and I feel as if the sun has gone into hiding. Darker moods bring other challenges that jump up to be noticed. Focusing on my problems, for example, saying, "Oh, I feel so ill...!", makes me feel worse, which brings me more of what I don't want. I breathe life into my problems by honouring them with my attention, much as if I were building a wall and trying to clamber over it at the same time. If when we feel ill or unhappy we might say instead, "I feel happy and well," the recovery of our optimism is much speedier. So, the occasional cough or sniffle becomes an opportunity to experiment with a different attitude.

Allow Life to Unfold

Allowing life to unfold is another very useful habit we can cultivate. This state of allowing works most agreeably when I accept that the Universe is entirely benign and constantly engineering the best outcome in every circumstance. We put our faith and commitment to the test when we work hard at our chosen projects. Perhaps we have spent a lifetime making challenging and difficult decisions. If, however, we find our path constantly strewn with boulders of difficulty, we may come to believe that the difficult path is more worthwhile, more real. It may take time to clamber over all the obstructions in our way and navigate ourselves back to a smoother path.

If we can accept that the Universe is constantly recalibrating our "satellite navigation" to bring us back to a place where we feel content, then we can observe "difficult" circumstances while doing our best to stay steady and keep moving towards the peace we are aiming for. As we grow older, we more obviously notice this progression and can agree, "I really have had the most amazing life. Many wonderful things have happened to bring me here today."

When I make the mistake of "searching" for miracles, for answers to my many anguished questions, feelings of inadequacy resurface so that I feel as if I have spent the last three – or thirty – years wandering across parched deserts of hopelessness where nothing flowers, where the best days of my life have departed, leaving me stranded, exhausted and alone; which is exactly how it feels at the time. *Searching* for anything, whether it be happiness, fulfilment, enlightenment, patience, wisdom or wads of cash, simply propels it away from us, as we canter after it screaming, "Come here!" Doesn't sound promising, does it?

Instead of erecting the Discovery of Happiness (or Miracles, or Serenity, or Peace or My Destiny) into My Next Big Project, I can make a small start by refusing to be blinded by the difficulties in everyday everything. Instead of dissecting all my problems at great length with anyone who will listen, I find that life is more rewarding when I allow silence a bit of room, let go and feel myself floating over the top of a problem, on my way to the next better thing.

Avoid Negative Situations

I avoid party poopers, doom-mongers and gossips on the lookout for the next titbit. Travellers whom I meet on the bus frequently eye my walking aid speculatively and ask, "What's the matter with you, then?" When I smile and reply, "I'm feeling absolutely fine, thanks!" or "It's a long story" (*which I would rather not share right now, if you don't mind*) they make a disappointed face and move to another seat. Yet, my response is neither rude nor dismissive. I don't enjoy swimming around in the victim mentality any more. It makes me unhappy and unwell.

Other people may enjoy dignifying their lives with a sense of how uniquely difficult everything is for them. They may even feel that life's difficulties are what define them and in many ways they may be right. Thoughts are creative, after all. Most of us living in more affluent parts of the world can afford to look more playfully at preoccupations we usually consider difficult and resist "arguing" with them. We don't want to rely on a sense of aggravation to get a buzz, do we?

Gentle optimism is more rewarding. Let us keep the peace and refuse to be railroaded by "painful reality", if only because we know that, in the midst of intentional peacefulness, miracles are emboldened to come out and play. If the Universe sees us smiling, do you not think it is pleased? Will not Life bless those who can encounter sorrow and setbacks and still smile at the end of the day? Miracles are drawn to us when our steady cheerfulness lights up the world with gentle welcome. So train your gaze on something positive and keep it there, whenever your mind threatens to descend into the slough of despond. Go within and reconnect with the joy of being present in every moment, while you sidestep the myriad taunts of the ego to become embroiled in complications that have no answer. Eventually, difficulties may be met as a small challenge, a mental and spiritual exercise to test our resolve. How much have we learned? Are we adept at dodging the spears of discomfort that Life throws at us?

Practise Forgiveness

When we are determined to focus on the positives in our lives – and there is always something we can feel grateful for – we are part of a process that, taking a longer view, aims to forgive everyone and everything we consider negative. Annoying events or persons and intractable situations can be released: as a frustrated, disabled woman, I can experiment with allowing more ease into my life by agreeing, "I now accept, love and bless my body." Whenever life saddens or frustrates me, I feel better taking a step back and saying, "I am grateful for the gifts I receive each day" or "I forgive and release this situation." I feel soothed. Even when our expressing forgiveness gives rise to emotions such as grief, regret or anger, allowing such emotions to surface and have expression is a wonderful step in healing. Blessing or forgiving any situation lets it go, which feels so relaxing.

"I forgive you," means different things. Perhaps the least helpful version translates as, "You were horrible to me – I was your victim for a while and I am going to make a martyr of you now (and maybe for the rest of your life, I'll see how that goes)." How many of us have said, "I forgive you," when we really mean, "I want you to feel guilty"? I know I have.

"I forgive you," may mean, "I am happy and whole now. Please stop grovelling as you are refuelling a grumble that I have been working hard to overcome. Please do not reignite my sense of grievance."

In its most life-affirming, joyful sense, "I forgive you" means, "I release you and bless you because nothing you do really hurts me." Blessing whatever happens – good and bad – strengthens my conviction that I always choose what I allow into my space. In the same way, I refuse to get caught up in the blame game. I come from a feeling of abundance in my good fortune that nothing and no-one can upset. How many of us have come so far that we can mean, "There is nothing to forgive"?

Martyrdom is not forgiveness, since that response would say, "You are killing me but that's okay, I don't count (as much as you do). (But I'm going to make you pay for this, sometime.)"

In the final analysis, self-interest is at the root of forgiveness and is the answer that finally ends the time-consuming and futile mind games around self-pity, grudges and resentment. It is not because you have done something wrong that I hope to forgive you: forgiveness and letting go clear away my shad-ows, confusion and stumbling blocks. In that way, I am being rather selfish, determined to keep my cheerfulness intact.

One winter evening while I was staying at my sister's house, I wrote in my journal:

> I woke in a good mood and was leafing through the book, *Why Forgive?* (3) in which many of the usual "you are so naïve" argu-ments are rehearsed by those of us who may be unwilling to forgive, or to use the power of quiet humility as the author suggests. I was

left thinking about the light of forgiveness that can break down seemingly immovable blocks that surround us and appear to weigh a ton (see *Happiness Matters*, pp. 4-5).

I was pondering the idea that when I forgive you, I set myself free. Spoken aloud, these words sounded a challenge, a gauntlet left lying…and gently picked up to give me another piece of the jigsaw... "Forgiveness confers the gift of innocence as soon as it is offered; and if we are both innocent *what is there to fear?*" If there is no fear, we are free to act happily as God may direct.

Express Gratitude

Strengthening our ability to overlook difficulties and practise forgiveness can bring remarkable new perspectives and health benefits. Deploying heartfelt affirmations – with which we are free to articulate every positive belief and outcome we hope or intend for ourselves – ultimately reframes the way we see ourselves, and helps us to recognize our good fortune and express our pleasure in it.

When we say with conviction, "I am so lucky!" then, whether we realize it or not, we are immediately on the lookout for ways in which this holds true in our lives; and, as if in response to our gratitude, our luck improves – so long as we can resist the urge to kill the blossoming of our fortune stone dead with arguments such as, "That's just a coincidence, too good to be true. I don't believe it!"

Expressing gratitude is like a diamond. It has so many facets that sparkle in sunlight. Once we start showing gratitude there is no stopping us – we notice miracles of our lives everywhere. We understand that when our daughter wants to play with us we are lucky and that when we have food on the table, we are blessed. Recognizing and expressing gratitude is all it takes. And once we start the ball rolling, we can see that our whole existence is simply a series of blessings. So no matter what else may be going on, keep saying thank you and offer a shrug of resignation for those bits you cannot understand. One day soon, it may become clearer what all the painful compromises are for.

Clear Out Personal Space

To emphasize our change in attitude, there is nothing like a good clear out of our personal effects. All our possessions gradually become saturated with old feelings and memories – clothes, photographs, dusty mementoes and souvenirs which lie lopsidedly on our bedside cabinet. Among the business suits and blouses there are bound to be items we have hardly worn, such as that elegant dress given to me as a graduation present twenty years ago which I have never felt able to pass on because that would be ungrateful, even though it pinches under the arms and the colour does nothing for me. It can finally leave my wardrobe and go to a better home, along with the wooden jumper rack in several pieces that my mother bequeathed, the book that my sister passed on with the instruction "not to throw it out" and the darling pink angora sweater my sweet husband bought for Christmas one year which is three sizes too small. I was charmed that he saw me as petite, but wearing it emphasized my wide shoulders and neck. Next time he wants to purchase something expensive for me, I will suggest that we choose it together.

Many material objects we cling to take up precious space in our homes and in our thoughts. Do we really want them? If the answer is no, then start an export habit to the second-hand shops, the summer fair or car boot sale. Rewrap an unwanted present for a friend. There will be no shortage of takers and you will have lots of lovely space into which your new dreams can move more easily. Let's face it: space comes at a premium these days and what are you paying your mortgage for? To store your mother's unwanted tea sets?

The amount we discard tends to be a measure of how much we desire change. When we don the apron and rubber gloves, we can take a little care not to barge through everything like a tank in a greenhouse. Unless we have hoarded stuff for forty years or feel imminently at risk from piles of newspapers collapsing on top of us, we can take it easy to begin with, until the conviction grows within that we are happy to clear away all this stuff, at last! Joyful decisions feel light and easy.

Sometimes Spirit will force our hand. Last summer we had an outbreak of clothes moths in our cupboards. So everything in there, a space which had not been dusted for over a decade, got cleared out, bagged or binned and hoovered very thoroughly. As a nudge to clear the atmosphere, it certainly worked.

Go to the Woods

Trees, which I adore, feature in many of my dreams. The easy sway of branches and leaves over my head calms my breathing. When I gaze up into the canopy of a large tree, watching the shimmering yellow and green light on leaves and examining every detail, I notice how patterns of beauty are repeated, over and over again until the senses are overwhelmed, swimming in never-ending beauty. Looking at such unconscious, dazzling splendour is very humbling and refreshing. Such beauty is simply waiting for us to notice and bathe our senses in.

If I can make time to go to my nearest woodland, I am always grateful and energized to have made the effort. I give thanks for tall, strong trunks, for hidden root systems raising earthy contours in the ground beneath my feet. I imagine a hidden multitude of crawling insects, the flies, bugs and beasties that scuttle and swarm unseen and which all contribute to making the woodlands vibrant, healthy and strong. I love to stand still and watch a while, until I realize how vast I am compared to a hoverfly; and how small, compared to the rising arms of love arching above me.

Asking the question, "What would you like me to know?" I sit against a trunk or walk peacefully and listen. Gradually an answer will arrive.

One night, fed up with the usual round of predictable tedium – entirely of my making, I now realize – I asked for help. I was feeling cut adrift, bored, sore and rather as if I didn't care about anything. More importantly, I wanted to know what I was here to do, so that I might have a focus for my energy and something to look forward to. The following dream sequence was the result.

> A ghost angel, that almost formed as I wished, resolved into an old man, dark and filled with wisdom and secrets. He was a messenger who came from an angel, to talk

to me. I remember he talked in a strange language. I was left with two pictures.

First, a lantern in the dark night, with a light hanging on the end of a cast-iron pole. A light that would not be blown out because it sat at home behind its sheltering glass cover. The light signalled endless strength and possibility, endless answers and happiness waiting peacefully to light up my pathway through the darkness. I didn't have a clue where I was going but I had the light and IT WAS ALL I NEEDED.

Then the old man dissolved and I saw a coat stand. Unusual, but as it turned out, an excellent pun. I went back later to reconsider this image and two things jumped out at me. First, getting rid of old habits – as in, old clothes; habit is an old-fashioned word for clothes. And this was reinforced by the idea of casting off old hang-ups. Things we would hang up on an old coat stand. If I can get rid of all the old stuff – which is as easy as leaving it there – the rest will follow.

IS THAT A COINCIDENCE?

Coincidence: "a chance occurrence of events, remarkable either for being simultaneous or for apparently being connected".

Collins English Dictionary. (4)

When we are in the process of remembering our power – a process which never ends – sooner or later we notice coincidences. Coincidences are two aspects that meet when we least expect them to. For example, you are thinking of a friend and they telephone; you need some bread and your neighbour comes to the door with left-over groceries, including a loaf of bread which she offers you because she is going on holiday; half a dozen of you are going out for dinner and you find an empty table in the crowded restaurant; I am looking for a pair of shoes in a particular make and the shop has one pair left in the right size; I need a parking space and there it is, right in front of the restaurant / concert hall / doctors' surgery.

Last year, I delayed sending my friend a Christmas card. Then I noticed an obituary for one of her other friends whom I had once met, and knowing that Alice does not read newspapers, I clipped it out and sent it to her with a card. She telephoned the following morning to tell me that she had been sitting at her desk to send a seasonal card to that friend, when she spied the postman coming through her front gate, carrying my letter with the obituary. She knew to send a letter of condolence instead.

Have you ever had a beautiful dream? I know you have. I bet it filled you with wonder, delight and amazement. Have you ever tried to tell anyone else about it? Eyes glaze over and yawns are stifled. It is not that our nearest and dearest are heartless or thoughtless; and it's not that dreams are dull; but it can be frustratingly difficult to convey the vividness and impact of a dream to another person, don't you think? "Coincidence" has a similar reputation.

We have all seen or heard, noticed or unearthed something personal to us, like a song playing on the radio that we "just happened" to be thinking about, or a melody with special significance. Maybe our prayers of last night have been answered with a letter we received the next morning; or we have a spark of an idea, a thought or an inspiration that arrives exactly when it is most needed.

A novel I was reading contained this now rather

clichéd advice based on an old Cherokee story. *There are two wolves in your life. One is joy, peace, serenity, kindness and acceptance. The other is sorrow, anger, unhappiness, negativity and hatred. Which one will grow strong? The one you feed...* I put down the book and went to make dinner. Switching on the radio, I heard Duran Duran's song, "Hungry like a Wolf", blaring out over the airwaves. It might not be my all-time favourite song, but that kind of connection can be electrifying, reminding us that we are part of a bigger, wider picture which is moving heaven and Earth, constantly, to bring us our best possible outcomes.

We can start with the biggest miracle of all. Our being here is a pretty amazing, mind-boggling piece of luck, wouldn't you say? Is our existence here a mere coincidence? Thinking about how many strands and twists of fate brought me to where I am today makes my head spin. Whatever rationalists say, the word "coincidence" really doesn't explain enough to me. But if there is no such thing as coincidence then what on Earth is happening?

Being a naïve sort of woman who likes to speak to God in all sorts of ways and who notices more and more nudges and hints these days, I tend towards the view that there is no such thing as mere happenstance. I prefer to see coincidence as Life's way of signalling or helping me, either to choose what I could enjoyably do now, or to make life easier whatever I might be doing. Sometimes, a coincidence acts as useful validation that we are on the right track, just as, when things are continually difficult or we are constantly exhausted, this may be a hint that we are moving in the wrong direction.

Hints we would tend to ignore or dismiss can more happily be accepted as a signal from Life reminding us of our constant connection with our most meaningful purposes. Reminders and hints are helpful, since we often fail to notice when an action or decision is in our best interests. If we get caught up in the emotion of a personal attachment, for example, or are seduced by someone who pays us attention, it can be extremely challenging to step back and say, "This is not working out…"

By sending us messages in dreams and with daily signals, Spirit reminds us that we are all understood and helped along a path that will give us greatest scope for expanding our horizons and living well. What we contribute to the world is important. We are each so precious to the success of the whole, that Life is very happy to send us prompts, thoughts and ideas to help smooth the path and make living more enjoyable. Instances such as these will be familiar to us all. Here are a few of my favourite examples.

I was wondering where I might get some sugar for pancakes that I decided to make and about an hour later a small parcel arrived in the post from my sister. Among other things, she sent some small packets of vanilla sugar. She had never sent them to me before and has never sent them again.

I needed a new pair of elbow crutches. The ones I was using were old, the stoppers slippery and dangerous. In order to obtain a new pair from the hospital I would need to set up an appointment with my GP, make the visit to see her, get a referral to the local hospital out of town, go to that appointment, all of which could take weeks. Alternatively, I could purchase a pair on-line. In any case, I sent off a clear request to the Universe for some new crutches and promptly forgot all about it. The very next day I "just happened" to be standing at the kitchen window when I saw our new downstairs neighbours throwing out two brand new elbow crutches that had been abandoned by a previous tenant. My husband rescued these for me.

We were on holiday having an early supper at a Highland resort when the rain started pelting down. We had not thought to bring our coats from the car which we had parked some distance away. I was wondering what we would do, so I asked for help, then enjoyed the rest of my meal. After we had finished and were leaving, it was still raining heavily. A covered golf buggy drew up alongside the entrance steps and the driver kindly offered us a lift back to our car, in style!

In the early days of being a writer, I was wondering where to go with my first book. I asked for reassurance that all was well. I had a dream in which I was about three inches high, squat and dark. I looked as if I would have been more at home in a tropical climate. Nevertheless, I had entered a race through a freezing, snowy landscape, running against a real ice man, who was thin, tall, edgy, cool and supremely engineered for success in the frozen north. Just the two of us; and looking from him to me and back again, there was no doubt who would win and who would sink into deep snow at the first step – me! Nevertheless, I set off and soon I was clutching a medal around my chest, as a reward for my decision to enter the race and give it my best efforts. And that is indeed how my dreams of being published got started. Thanks to the help of readers and friends, I secured a coveted first place with an on-line writers' community and obtained a professional review of my work. These efforts were pivotal in securing my future publishing success.

For me, getting published was never going to be a logical, rational undertaking during which I would weigh up my chances and decide to go ahead. Since the odds against a new writer succeeding are so great, logic would tell me to go back to bed and forget the whole thing. Persisting with the dream despite astronomical odds was an act of faith: writing is simply what I do. I woke happy from this dream and told my husband about it. *Later that day* I was idly thinking that if I was serious about this publishing lark it might be a good idea to learn more about how the process works, so I retrieved my copy of the *Writers' and Artists' Yearbook* (5) and my hand chanced upon an article in the eight-hundred-page volume which contained nuggets of advice such as, "Unsolicited submissions (unflatteringly referred to as 'the slush pile') are the least likely to be taken up for publication". That night, still asking for help, I got another nudge, *You haven't been listening. We* ARE *speaking to you!* It was a real Eureka Moment!

I realized that Spirit must know a great deal about piles of slush by the side of the road and must be helping me find a path through them. After my dream of the night before, s/he made sure I picked up the *Yearbook* and read about slush-piles. And so I became convinced that my efforts would be for a purpose and that all was being guided and taken care of. In the spooky halls of happenstance, only I can know how far that particular set of circumstances went towards giving me the proof I sought. Our private wisdom slots together, for our eyes alone and ultimately for our benefit.

So…if you would like some help – big or small – ask cheerfully, then wait and see. Above all, resist the urge to splutter, "But that's impossible!" when a solution presents itself. "That must surely be a coincidence…" we say, and let the miracle pass us by. We automatically issue these killer sentences on our joy, without realizing what we are doing. Catch yourself next time and say thank you instead.

IS IT A DREAM OR IS IT REAL?

Here is a dream meditation which Spirit sent one morning. I woke in a state of floating bliss the likes of which I have never experienced before or since. Lingeringly, I understood that we help ourselves when we deploy our thoughts wisely. We are each inherently creative and powerful. We may use this meditation whenever we would like more light, relaxation and confidence.

MEDITATION on MATTER

GOOD FOR: anxiety, depression, sadness, when overstretched, for tiredness, loss of focus, bad energy, sleeplessness, obsessions, fear of failure, worry about the future, thinking too much.

Imagine that you are lying on a table, couch or a big bed. The room is warm and filled with comforting, gentle light and shadows. There are tall, all-seeing spirits and angels around the bed. As you feel any negative feeling come into your head, imagine that it is understood, bandaged and blessed, so that the ache in that part is soothed and removed. Every part of every ache and sorrow or failing which inhabits any part of you is recognized, bandaged and blessed with a laying on of hands. As you recognize and surrender each of the pains, frets and worries that you carry, it is understood with infinite compassion and patience, smoothed away with love, bandaged with infinite patience. Surrender to the care that is ministered and understand that the well of compassion being shared is infinite.

When the whole body is well bandaged – as it will be – there comes the transformation; for all at once there rises from the form on the table a myriad of swirling, bright, colourful lights, leaving the body. Escaping through the heart, the breath, or the eyes, all colours reunite above the body. They dance free, light and unencumbered, weightless and full of joy. Feel the light. Feel the colours, the freedom. Feel the limits of body falling away and dissolving. See behind you a pile of broken bandages; and before you a luminous and glorious pattern of unique and unspeakable beauty that is your own brilliance, dancing free at last, from the constraints and heaviness of our usual lives. The beautiful patterns of deep, vibrant, vivid colours make you dance and sing and clap your hands for joy. No weights, no thoughts, no limitations – just floating bliss and beauty. That is you.

Then, begin to notice for a short moment little, metallic plates of matter being attracted to your dancing spirit. These are thoughts, the limitations and intrusions of logic. Each thought, materializing as a detachment from the beautiful swirl, is like a small piece of flat shrapnel, that attaches like a shell to the outside of the spirit. Each tiny piece is evidence of a thought limitation, since, as the thoughts build up, they will form a shell over and around the spirit. See the pull of your thinking and what it attracts to you: plates of metal and rigidity in mind and body.

Move away from this picture of understanding, out again into the bliss of being unencumbered. Remember that feeling. Understand, finally, that:

- Thoughts are matter

- Matter is magnetic
- What you think on, attracts its like in material form
- Thoughts are magnetic
- We are creative beings
- ONLY SPIRIT IS REAL
- ALL ELSE IS ATTRACTED AND CREATED, ATTRACTED AND CREATED
- WE START AS SPIRIT
- WE CAN ESCAPE
- WE ARE LOVED, ALWAYS WE ARE LOVED
- ONLY LOVE IS REAL

Whether I find myself in a state of needing and questioning, or whether I have decided to be calm and more deliberately pray and ask for help, I find the early morning rewarding. Filled with peaceful optimism and energy and more receptive to help, while awake, I can reach places that feel very dreamlike. And, as if making the most of the opportunity to communicate, Spirit takes the opportunity of my relaxed state to drop information into my head.

My husband worries constantly about his work. One morning he was more worried than usual and I fretted because I did not know what I could say or do to comfort him. Immediately, Spirit stepped in and sent a picture of a hopping bird, about the size of a sparrow, whose shiny black plumage was streaked with gold. The bird was hopping on a fireplace, trapped behind a fireguard, jumping up and down on peats or coals that were heating up, smoking ominously. On closer inspection it was easier to notice that the bird's natural plumage was golden, though it had been turned black with the gradual overlay of sticky soot. Soot on its feathers blended with the dark bricks of the fireplace and as a result, the bird had been overlooked. Any moment now, the fire was going to take hold and flames would flare up, leaving the bird with nowhere to go.

Watching from my place at the side of the room, I knew what might happen but I could not reach the fire, because my legs felt as heavy as sandbags and I could not move forward, though I understood all the risks that the bird faced by remaining where it was, hopping frantically up and down on the spot and getting nowhere. If I could move, I could lift the fireguard away and help the bird to safety or freedom. I could do this and part of me understood that this was in my power. This was what I might do to help.

When I tried to tell my husband what I had seen, he mumbled something and went back to sleep. Despite feeling a bit frustrated, here was another lesson: since I find it hard to explain pictures like these convincingly to other people, they must be sent mostly for my benefit. That picture helped me to understand what my husband was experiencing but could not explain. Therefore, messages and dreams are mainly intended to help me to be more sympathetic or more relaxed, not to persuade my husband or bully him towards a course of action that I may think is obvious. Instead of nagging, I can push forward with my own projects, which may one day come to fruition and so offer my husband hope of changing his difficult circumstances. Seeing and appreciating his predicament has indeed been the best incentive I could ask for, to work diligently on my own projects. Until he makes changes which he has chosen for himself, doing my own work as sincerely as I can is the best contribution I can offer him.

On another occasion, when something of my husband's behaviour was irritating and I prayed, "Please could you make Eddie stop?" immediately the answer came back, "NO! Ask instead for help to relax!" The help I am sent is intended to help me decide what I can do, not to cajole someone else or force their hand.

Making time and space to enjoy a visualization, I may find myself strolling among trees beside a waterfall or swimming, then dressing in a beautiful robe and walking through gardens where sweet-smelling blossoms wave in the wind, reminding me that happiness is everywhere. There, along a path, is a bench placed beside healing lavender bushes and overlooking the sea. Refreshing, salty breezes heighten my senses. I may meet a person with a message for me, someone from family, a new friend… It could be anyone. We talk and share. We are content, embraced by the light around us and the life that lives at peace with us wherever we cast our eyes. Birds hover overhead and I can witness that life brims with joy and promise. In such settings, visualizations may take on their own momentum.

For example, one morning I woke and consciously focused on feelings of release, speaking words of blessing aloud: "I am indeed blessed and all around me the world is filled with blessings. I am at peace and all is peaceful." After agreeing with the good in my life in this way for about five minutes, I felt very warm, relaxed and certain. I continued, "We are Spirit in a body, eternal spirit with the power of all Spirit to summon to ourselves our goodness, our desires. No desire is overlooked or left behind. All is acceptable in the sight of Spirit and all my desires are drawn to me by my certainty. There is no shame, no loss, only acceptance of my power and freedom."

Power pulses through us, hopefully pushing us beyond old constraints and worn-out routines. In declaring my peace and certainty, I found the dream moving ahead gladly, pleased to be able to share something new. I found myself at the trade entrance of a supermarket, where the swing doors moved forward easily, opened by my certainty. I got a trolley and was filling it with whatever I wanted. The first thing I asked for was a juicy melon, then a mango, then some apples, some zingy oranges, then flowers and more fruit: refreshment for a thirsty spirit, perhaps? At first, the freedom to choose whatever I wanted was paralyzing, though it gradually dawned on me that yes, I was free to choose whatever I desired. Gradually, the doors of my desire opened and all my choices came tumbling out: a holiday in the sun, good food to eat, friendship and laughter, help with the housework, free time to relax and be happy. As I was going round and choosing, in the store the shelves were getting tidier and more organized, more beautiful and ordered with so many things to choose from: flowers in bunches as far as the eyes could see; plane tickets to fly to anywhere in the world lying there neatly ordered and ready to pick up; exotic food, lovely fragrances. Everything became more and more beautiful as my certainty came into focus.

As I refined my present desires I also noticed my usual obsessions losing their iron grip on my thoughts. Old, well-worn preoccupations around not having enough money, being downtrodden or failing in my relationships were at the back of the queue somewhere, while I was drawn towards activities that were fun, refreshing and rejuvenating. Everywhere, refreshment was offering boundless energy and the self-belief to persist with my hopes.

When I got to the checkout desk, I was allowed to take home all my purchases and I was given a cheque for their value. Checkout, cash desk. Wow. The Universe has a wonderful, generous sense of humour. This sequence was great fun and very easily it proved that in choosing whatever fills us with joy, the Universe falls into order behind our choices gladly. Choices made with our happiness at their heart bring brightness, ease and fun. So we have nothing to lose and everything to gain from honouring our deepest desires.

> Another picture came to me as I woke one morning: a little dark man, short, squat and strong, a wild man, is standing beside a tall, dark tree at the heart of the forest. At the back of the tree, away from staring eyes, hidden among creepers and in the knots of the bark, is carved a sinuous ladder which reaches right up to the top of the tree. It feels like part of the tree, a willing part, not harming it at all. The man is pleased. He can

climb the tree nimbly and safely any time he wishes, right to the top where he can select and eat the choicest fruits from the high branches. From the topmost parts of the tree he can see his heavens.

LISTENING

I believe that a nameless faith sustains us throughout life. From infancy I knew that life was beautiful and that each day was magical. I didn't need a Sunday-school teacher telling me what it said in the Bible. I knew what I knew: that we are all precious and have our part to play in the unfolding of the miracle that happens when we live together peacefully.

Messages we receive are not only about grand events or lofty ambitions. They hold reassurance about all our daily preoccupations, small details that we would like filled in, as well as excellent insight into personal relationships, the state of our career plans and finances, even what foods we could steer clear of. Since all help makes it easier to stay focused and cheerful, it is valuable. Whatever time we take to record dreams is well invested. And as we write about them, our dreams become more real. Our intention and actions in anchoring dream pictures in writing, gives them space in our reality so that we get used to listening. Intrigued, we forget to be cynical; and the more we listen, the more help we receive.

This is one of the very first messages I remember receiving and understanding. I was maybe fifteen years old. I have carried this picture around with me like a talisman, never quite believing it, yet knowing that it is true for all of us.

I am at an open-air market and I have clasped in my hand my small, palm-sized purse which is decorated with sinuous and beautiful patterns of yellows, browns and oranges. It looks and feels like shimmering snakeskin – alive. I am scrubbing away at this purse – trying to polish up my sense of worth? – with steel wool, trying to buff it up to a shine and the harder I scrub, the more scratched and dull becomes the surface. My hard scrubbing propels the purse from my hand, where it lands in the mud, exposing the other side, which is shiny, smooth, sleek and vividly beautiful. The contrast it offers with all my scrubbing illuminates my understanding at once! There is no need for this hard work. Instead, let go, relax and let yourself shine in natural beauty. There is nothing you have to do.

I knew what this message was saying. And so, from that small beginning it became ever harder to ignore guidance, which became increasingly insistent as time passed. Unfortunately, for many years I was lost in the struggle. I took so many wrong turns and made so many mistakes that my life began to resemble a shattered teacup that has been dropped, the pieces collected up and glued together countless times. No matter how often I hurtled to the floor, someone somewhere seemed to want me to live and lovingly held my pieces together.

One major cause of my unhappiness was a belief that I was alone. I stopped seeing any miracles around me and believed in difficulty, hardship, heartache and sorrow. Not surprisingly, that was the best I could come up with at the time – free will, magnetism and cause and effect can be painful, when their power is twisted in unproductive ways.

During a long and painful decade in my earlier working life, I had a recurrent dream in which I was driving my red mini. Hurtling or sliding all over the place, it had no steering wheel, or the door handles were missing, or it got stuck in the mud. Naturally, I was frightened, though now I understand that Spirit was telling me my career was out of my control, beyond me, going downhill or with no sense of direction. I had no handle on the situation. Really, how dim can you be? Repeatedly, my minders urgently tried to set me on the right path, sending me constant and graphic reminders of my discomfort, my lack of control, my unsuitability for the job. (I never got to drive a wonderful car!) I don't usually admit to having recurrent dreams – which seem a bit too incredible – though this theme has kept me company for years and still returns occasionally. If I had listened more closely and acted on the guidance that I was being offered, how might my life have been different? How much pain might I have avoided?

It was when pictures regularly started to come in which were slow, shimmering and vivid, brightly coloured and stark that I could no longer dismiss them. I could not ignore the knowledge that I was being guided. My prayers began to feel less random; the answers I was being sent were so interesting, clever and amusing, that my cynicism lessened and eventually left me. I felt so intimately understood and occasionally have woken hearing a voice that has gently but emphatically set me right.

One evening I was upset about some item that had been dominating the news. I prayed about it and as I did, felt myself becoming more and more upset. Earnest and detailed were my requests. Endlessly I felt my yearning for a happy outcome and – in the midst of my angst – sent up despairing pleas, thinking that my fervour would strengthen my request. If prayer helped, then I was not going to be called a slacker! At intervals I begged for help. All night this continued, as I felt myself caught up in the drama. My dreams were fitful, despairing. Towards morning I fell into an exhausted stupor and in that magical interval between dozing and waking, when we are best caught off-guard, I fell asleep. Perhaps moments later, I was woken by a gentle voice which spoke kindly, "I do appreciate a good prayer. But I do not know how I am to answer it, if I cannot get a word in edgeways!"

More recently, after a long time of waiting for something, I challenged the early morning by declaring, "My life is a desert" and the reply came straight back, "It is a land flowing with milk and honey!" Messages like these certainly pack a punch.

How many of us avoid quietness and listening, or praying in our own way? We are shy to ask because we think that "It is never that easy" or "I am too busy" or "God cannot be interested in listening to me" or "the angels have far more important things to do…"

None of these excuses matters much. It is easy to pray and to ask. It is easy to listen. We are invited and indeed encouraged to place our concerns on the table, because, free will being what it is, if we don't ask, we don't get. I bet my life that the Universe aka the Sexy Suit in the Sky enjoys granting our wishes.

If the word *prayer* sets your teeth on edge or brings to mind the hard-bitten preachers of old, you are not alone. One of the biggest problems that the

Universal Organizer has, is that we have already told ourselves what s/he is all about and the devotional words we use, such as prayer, *Jesus Christ, God, Heaven* and so forth, with which we attempt to explain our spiritual beliefs, are loaded with cultural baggage and misunderstandings.

Perhaps instead of *prayer group* I can use the phrase *optimism circle*. Would that help? When we send out our dearest intentions and our deepest wishes, Her Upstairs has some excellent material to work with. So I challenge you to forget about being self-conscious and give the Great Dressmaker a chance. Instead of offering your poor, grey, miserable and shabby scraps, try sending up some of your most vibrant, colourful, cheerful, funny, foot-tapping, waltzing, free-wheeling, singing hopes. Have a great time digging out all your real desires and give yourself a party.

I used to make collections of worthless things: fruit wrappers printed on tissue paper or pencil shavings in a little plastic box, complete with the broken pieces of blue, purple and green lead that fell out of the pencil sharpener. Goodness knows what I was going to do with my pile of shavings, but, in its minimalist way, I thought it was beautiful. The material worthlessness of my collections appealed to me: I saw then, and still see now, the value in resurrecting beauty from discards. I used to admire the shimmer in flies' wings. I could see iridescence in there which looked like God's infinite tenderness. But were my modest ambitions reflecting a lack of self-belief? Was I worth leftovers and small oddments? It seemed a shame to throw these away; and for some reason, when it came to finding the bigger beauties in bright and sweet-scented roses, in paints and landscapes, shawls or clothes, my courage failed, as if total beauty might make me cry so hard I would never stop.

Though I tried to tiptoe past the really big, bright colours which had comforted me as a young child, reassurance was never far away. As a teenager seriously stalled in dull blues and greys, I dreamed I could see up into a very high sky. Up over my head, away in the dizzying distance, I perceived a delicately clouded ceiling, painted white and blue like a Vermeer masterpiece. Above soaring steeples, up in the heavens, the roof of the world was tiled. This picture reminds me that although we are not always aware of it, everything in life fits and takes its place in making a beautiful picture. If any tile is missing, if any piece of the jigsaw is lost, it leaves a hole. The sheer wonder of soaring height and delicate loveliness of this image helped me.

Until vibrant dreams came along to remind me I was worth more than leftovers, I dawdled rather out of sight, hoping to be overlooked, yet yearning to be understood. Dream beauty reminded me how much

I adore deep blues, vibrant reds and yellows. To this day, I remain forgetful of beauty, music, good food and fresh air, but in place of loss, I am more able to remember that every moment is a blessed opportunity to rediscover wonder. Colour and beauty offer spiritual refreshment, food for the soul, reaching and restoring parts of ourselves that cannot otherwise be satisfied. We need beauty in our lives, as a bird needs air in which to sing, or a dolphin needs waves to hold him up as he plays.

I urge you to go outside, look for something beautiful and remember why you like it. Fetch into your life bright poppies and peonies, autumn leaves, music, birdsong, blue sky, sunsets, soaring trees, a beautiful lawn of green bordered with cheering orange, the sounds of people having a good time, a delicious meal, a smile and a hug from someone you love. When I allow my heart to soften, the miracle of living shows itself in every beautiful moment.

If you think other people matter more, or if you routinely expect that you should postpone your pleasure until later; if you fear ridicule, or you fear you will be overwhelmed by beauty, remember – the miracles we notice in our lives are essentially a private affair. You need not worry that the whole world is going to laugh at you if you see an angel in the clouds. You don't have to tell them. Your understanding of God's beauty and how it meets your life is for you alone to appreciate and cultivate quietly.

DREAM PICTURES

Life has never once agreed with us while we have been persuading ourselves that miracles have to be difficult, you realize. Nor does Life agree that miracles happen only to famous people or are reserved for the really major issues of the day. We think that miracles must inevitably involve crossing the Red Sea without the aid of a raft, feeding three thousand people with a couple of scones or bringing someone back to life. We set ourselves such ludicrously high standards in miracles, just as we do with other aspects of success, that we can never see our humble selves having anything to do with them.

But you know I am going to say it doesn't have to be like that. Miracles are big and small, quiet and grand. They come in all shapes and sizes. A friend who phones me to reorganize some meeting, may have been prompted to do so because Life knows I have a double booking that day, even though I have forgotten. The coming together of small chances may be working towards a happy outcome.

Our dreams can be portals to wisdom and magic, like doors opening on a world that hides behind the light. If you would like to see more clearly what is on the other side of the door, it is helpful to keep a pad with a pen by your bed. Even better, purchase an elegant lined jotter in which all the pages are fixed or sewn in, so that you can't cheat and tear out passages or notes that you think are pointless. I am quick to defend "meaningless, useless scribbles" that we think we should tidy away into the dustbin. Small snapshots and pictures are as important as longer sequences and often more valuable: a single picture is easy to remember and can reveal so many messages, which are only obvious later or with the passage of time. So collecting them together in a journal will keep everything safely in one place for you to rediscover and refer back to.

Decorate the cover of your private book with beauty and love and then write whatever occurs to you, whatever messages you wake up with. Draw, write or make lists and collect dreams, insights, symbols, poems, advice, even nudges, words or names you mutter at two in the morning. I find that early morning communications are the clearest. My mind is more open and receptive, more relaxed after sleep.

Our souls are our larger selves in spirit, who love us to be happy. To that end, they are constantly reminding us of all the ways in which we can find ever greater fulfilment. Accepting guidance is like plugging ourselves in to universal energy. To provide reassurance and help lift away heaviness, our souls often communicate using symbols. When I see a picture which is vivid, unusual or filled with puns, I know that my soul, or Source, is sending a message. I receive single pictures filled with meaning, which carry the most amazing, inspiring, life-altering revelation. Filled with excitement, I record what I can remember and wait for the next step, reassured that answers and understanding will come when the time is right and I am ready to hear and accept them. As we become accustomed to trusting, we appreciate that our direct requests are always heard and answered, which in itself is immensely reassuring.

We can each learn how to interpret these signs and dreams for ourselves, in a process which moves us ever closer to soul prompts and to accepting help to reach our higher goals. Our soul keeps careful watch over our life purposes and will do everything it can to help us attain them.

In the early hours of the morning, sometimes I will receive a name or a nudge and, complacent that I will remember it and can safely wait until morning, I roll over and go back to sleep. Of course, by the time eight o'clock arrives I have usually forgotten the specifics and then, oh, how I wish I had made the small effort to switch on the bedside light and write. Written out on the page, a whole array of small meaningful details is much harder to dismiss. Shorthand puns, metaphors and jokes, insights gained over a period can mature with time, slowly being pieced together to form a most valuable personal dictionary. As your journal is for you, only you need ever read it.

Whether you are good at recalling your dreams or tend to forget them as soon as you wake up, every dream is effective at some level. The soul remembers everything – each moment, feeling and circumstance – and always steers us towards our highest good. However, our active involvement in a process of remembering, recording and reflecting, reminds us that in our earthly endeavours we are co-creators with Spirit, as well as sharpening our focus and acting as vital reassurance during periods of personal uncertainty or growth.

Using mere words, I can never do justice to the complexity and richness of the symbolism or the clues we can unearth. I can't do that for you. In your journal, you can and will collect unique understanding. Years, even decades later, I still recall many of the most vivid pictures I have received. I am continually astonished at what I see again, when, after days and weeks or even months and years, I reread what I may have jotted down in passing, while a nudge or a picture was fresh in my mind. Over the years, there is scope for real transformation.

In the meantime, I offer the following suggestions which I hope you may find useful. If my ideas do not feel right for you, please ignore them. Entries are taken directly from my dream journal, with little alteration.

Portals and archways

Archways = inspiration, hope, our connection with divine guidance and moving forward; a new phase of life; awareness of advice being offered. Consider your dream picture. How high is your archway? What is it made of? Marble, wood, cotton, cloth, fibre, tree arches, clouds, rainbows, water, stone or leaves? Each substance carries feelings and meaning for you. Is an entrance or archway carved in heavy, weathered stone with fissures and cracks? Is it solid and reliable, or ethereal and fleeting? Is it an archway of optimistic, cleansing water, or a downpour drenching your dreams? Is someone archly pissing on you from a great height? How do you feel about this image? In the way it is framed, each picture discloses secrets for you.

Rainbows perhaps merit a special mention. One evening I sent up a prayer, asking for forgiveness for something I had done, which, while not shocking or bad, was getting me down. I closed my eyes and asked carefully and clearly to be forgiven. When I opened my eyes, one of the biggest, brightest and clearest rainbows I have ever seen was hanging from a clear blue sky, right outside the window, over my head.

Another time, I was working on a project for which lots of outside support was vital. Rather doubting the strength of that support, which had caught me by surprise, I had a dream about a great ribbon of rainbow-coloured cloth, fastened to a bridge near my home. The ribbon of cloth soared up into the sky, in several great archways. It may have been a ribbon sewn from cloth, but it was holding firm on a strong clip. A rainbow sends a message that I am being listened to, my prayers are heard and I am being answered.

Doors

Doors = outgrowing present situations; going forward; awareness of and willingness to change; making choices; growing up and growing older; discovery, excitement and enlightenment. Are you searching? Are you trying to get through a door? Is your door small, clogged up with earth, decay, roots, darkness or sorrow? Have you lost the key? Is there an obvious lock, or is the door smooth and impenetrable? Are you happy or relieved as you try to push through? Is resistance heavy, or does the way forward clear easily? Is there light on the other side? What are the colours like? Vibrating, solid, luminous? Shaded, heavy, clouded?

Cars

Cars = our self, our inner space, our lives, our ambitions and feelings, our private lives, our way forward. Is your car spacious, too big or too small? Lots of room to manoeuvre, or cramped? What colour is it? Is the paintwork bright and shiny, or dull and neglected? Is the bodywork rusty, filled with holes? Is paintwork scratched or buffed to a shine? Your windscreen wipers may be on or off, broken or hanging loose. The wipers may be cleaning the window or sitting, blocking or scratching the view. Is your vision going forward clear, or obscured by dirt? Lights and horn may be working or broken. Can you find the door handle? Are you locked in? Do you have a full tank of petrol or are you running on empty? Do you have a steering wheel or does your car career out of control so you have no grip on your circumstances? Are you being driven or is someone driving you? Back seat driver? Where are you going? Is the weather fine or cloudy? Raining, snowing, icy cold, windy? Are you travelling downhill or up a steep incline? Either of these could mean difficulty. Uphill = struggle and obstacles; downhill = out of control, slipping or veering off course. Are you on the flat? = dull; or in a marsh = bogged down? Is it raining = are you unhappy?

Bicycles

Can be a message about the state of our ambitions and careers; our chosen pathways. I had a dream about a tall man on a bicycle. The bike was child- sized to his large frame and very rusty. He was trying to ride the bike and to fix the rusted chain that kept falling off. He kept pedalling, but the handlebars banged his knees with every turn of the wheels, which were bent and warped. The bike was a wreck, a write-off. So, the man stopped what he was doing and stood tall. In doing so, he seemed to grow even taller. The bike fell away and disappeared, as the path became very clear and straight, very smooth, with no obstacles. Stepping away, the man's strides grew longer, until with giant steps he moved rapidly forward towards a new life. This is a very clear dream of the state of a career. Stop trying so hard and move away from a difficult, frustrating life. Leave it alone and walk away. The message is clear and unambiguous.

Trees

Trees = self, self-expression, rootedness. Their height and form reflect personality and type. Is a tree small and compact, or broad, standing solitary in a clearing or crowded in with many others? Tall, thin and unbalanced, or mature, well-rooted and soaring high? What season is it and what colours do you see? Are the roots deep or shallow; are they stable or do they rock back and forth as the wind blows? Are you standing or sitting beneath a tree which cuts out the light – is someone dominating you? Are you in a crowded forest, or do you have room to stretch your arms and your creativity wide?

Contrasting dreams about trees can show how much knowledge lies waiting to be unearthed.

Feeling troubled by a picture of a rocking tree, I have been unsure how I will stabilize it. This tree is tall and slender, but unstable, since its roots sit atop a very large, hard boulder that it cannot escape. Whichever way the boulder rocks, the tree sways, trapped above it. Tree roots reach down just far enough to brush the earth tantalizingly. Each time an anchoring might grow, the boulder rolls unsteadily, so that no roots are ever established which would help to stabilize or plant the tree firmly.

There is another tree which finds itself holding on precariously at the very edge of a deep precipice, clinging on to the edge of flat earth, beneath which the ground falls away sharply. In a leap of understanding I realize that I can take matters into my own hands, in my dreams as well as my waking life. Right then, I decide to escape my instability and uncertainty by somersaulting straight into the void, a handstand roll down the hill to free myself. When I have righted myself – another pun – I see that I am standing in a gentle ravine, in water, in a wood, where I can be gentle, sylph-like and happy at last. I am now a small native tree, a hardwood – strong – hazel or silver birch, but I feel at home here, well anchored and peaceful and from this place I have room to expand and grow upwards again.

Lately I had been moving away from the metaphor of trees because I felt their root-edness was unhelpful, unmoving and stuck. I should have known better. Before waking this morning I was gifted the picture of a beautiful, broad tree, tall and strong. I am reminded that the constituent parts of any tree move a great deal. Yes, the roots are planted very firmly and deeply and that is good as it allows a tree to flourish and to draw nourishment from the dark soil, itself a metaphor for our less happy experiences. It is good when roots are well anchored, deep and holding strongly.

But leaves are always moving, as are swaying branches. And the seeds! Seeds can travel great distances by many different means: wind, water, carried by animals. They fall and are taken away to start other good trees. Seeds are an excellent symbol, wrapped up in the notion of gentle, peaceful exchange, growth and discovery.

Gardens and fields

Fields and gardens = states of possibility and growth; courage and willingness to change; ideas and opportunities.

I recall a vivid dream I had when I was younger, of walking along a high wall, doing a tricky balancing act with the aid of a long pole, but in the end falling off and down into an urban garden. The lawn on which I landed flat on my back was very small and the walls closed me in, though the grass I lay on was very fresh, green and comfortable. It would be very easy to lie there and do nothing. I could stay there for a long time, sleeping perhaps, or looking up at the bright blue sky and watching the passing clouds, but there was little room to move… The walls were very high, so escape from here would be very difficult… What should I do?

The dream is about how I felt at the time: closed

in, bricked up, in a seemingly easy situation, a "cushy number" but in fact difficult, with no room to manoeuvre or any change of position. Pinned on my back = helpless?

In happier circumstances, I dreamed of a large field of bright yellow wheat with a wide path cut around the edge. The gate to the field was a simple wooden construction, pulled open easily and with little to stop anyone entering. I knew I had permission to go in and do whatever I wished. Would I sleep in the summer sun, lying around the edge, where it was warm and comfortable, or would I consider what to do with the crop? Whose crop was it? It could be mine. At the height of summer – at this time of my life – it was ripe and easy to reach. Golden wheat suggests a bright future, nourishment and abundance, fruitful possibility. I could have it if I wished, but then, I might have to put in some work to gather it up, store it and use it. I might even want to think about what next season's crop might be. The choice was mine.

Insights don't arrive neatly parcelled up and straightforward. Our souls, being far greater and wiser than we know, understand only too well that if they told us everything straight, we might not hear. If messages are too directly instructive, we might resist, so instead, we are sent dreams which match our current understanding and take us a step further forward. If there is some urgency, we can usually feel it keenly: that red dream I had about the toilet was direct, frightening and overflowing with meanings that I could not ignore.

Like pictures, dream textures and the feelings they arouse are all personal and instructive. Dreams remind us of the state we are in, perhaps suggesting that now is the time to address a problem we have been avoiding, or to follow up an opportunity we have let slide. If a matter needs urgent attention, a picture may be frightening, claustrophobic, amusing or ludicrous, to point out how far the situation has moved away from what is ideal. A dream my husband had about an aardvark being interviewed for a job comes to mind. Here is another message that came in an unusual way.

> As I was walking to the school pick-up, right in front of me on the canal, a most unusual sight: a mother moor hen, her legs and feet splayed wide apart on a small island of tufted grasses shorn away from the bank. On this precarious island in the middle of the wind-blown water of our shallow canal, where longboats and day trippers are routine, the mother hen is making a home she thinks is safe from feral cats on the bank and from foxes lurking. But her efforts are futile, as very soon another bank of canoes with

wide oars will disturb her. Her safety is an illusion and all her work is for nothing. Is this a reminder to me that housework is better left aside for now? The daily graft has no permanence, after all. Perhaps I would be better to do other things and put my energies elsewhere. As my friend Elaine commented on seeing the scene, "One small canal boat and she is doomed!"

Animal totems

Which is your favourite animal? For many years, I was very fond of the duck-billed platypus; later I would have chosen an elephant; then I settled upon the giraffe. These days I gravitate towards the wolf padding faithfully across the ground and his counterpart the eagle which soars through the sky.

It occurs to me that the platypus is an animal made of an apparently confusing mix of parts. To look at it, you might think it had been fashioned out of bits and pieces. But it works well and does its own thing quite happily. At the time, that felt like me: all at sixes and sevens, unusual – and with a noxious kick! – but functioning well enough.

The elephant moves very slowly and could be accused of thinking too hard. Ponderous, determined and perhaps rather introverted, the responsibilities of life weigh it down. That was me later, all plodding and unsure, walking carefully and with a heavy weight around my shoulders.

The giraffe has a big heart and long, delicate legs that take it up and away from the cares of Earth. Perhaps a little unsure on its feet and ungrounded, it seems to rise too close to heaven, so it may appear to be impractical and given to shy introspection. All these animals have a special place in my heart. I notice how much I have identified with each of them during different stages of life.

Nowadays I happily accept the wolf as a favourite. In the loyal, physically active wolf pack which has a lot of ground to cover, I am accepted and work as part of a team. I am more able to allow others to extend help and to embrace the success which comes from teamwork. That feels liberating and very strong. A good firm base near the ground, aligned with greater determination to persist and not give up when the path becomes more difficult. From success, we build more success together. But taken too far, over-reliance on the pack can lead to the imbalance of dependence, making me incapable of thinking for myself, which can produce feelings of being vulnerable and depressed.

Right on cue, above all the animals soars the eagle, whose unquestioning strength and peace is available to me when I need to let go of everyday concerns that threaten to become too dominant or leave me stuck in the ground, unable to decide or move. The eagle represents quiet strength and unquestioning assistance, as well as higher perspective and the detachment that comes from being at a distance. The eagle decides for himself, as he must, being a solitary creature who lives remote from others. His great strength of purpose and single-mindedness remind me that I can be alone with God. In that state, I can act powerfully, decisively and for the furtherance of my own plans. I can – and ultimately I must – make my own decisions and discover the courage and resources to live with the consequences.

When I asked who my guides were, I received a very clear flash of an eagle, brown and white colouring; big, independent and strong. I have seen it before, the eagle. It is very private and determined: the necessary counterbalance to my softness, my yielding and giving all the time, this feeling I have of being stretched. Conversely, when I become over-reliant on the eagle, I become isolated and lonely. The trick is to balance the eagle with the wolf.

I also find comfort with the horse, which for me strikes a wonderful balance between strength and sensitivity. With the horse as helper, I can take great strides. Being that bit higher off the ground than the wolf, I can gallop ahead. However, there are times when I still need to be careful: A horse can become ill very suddenly and in unexpected ways, so I may need to pace myself, or act with caution. I have seen lots of horses in my dreams, flying, galloping and taking me forward as I cling excitedly to the mane.

It is a simple, almost childlike question to ask, "Now, what is my favourite animal?" You may ask, make a note in your journal and remember other connected thoughts from the past. Note these too and ask for clarity. Who knows what your chosen favourites reveal about your strengths and weaknesses? Do we feel an affinity with particular animals because their weaknesses and strengths feel familiar?

DUET WITH THE LIGHT WORLD

Our heavy Earth balances on a delicate axis and plots a careful course between extremes: extremes of darkness and light, cold and heat, humidity and aridity. To the untrained eye it may look rather rough and ready, yet we are beginning to realize that the smallest variation, for example in ambient temperatures, can have far-reaching consequences. There are so many variables that need to be kept in balance and the process by which the natural world sustains life is, in many ways, mirrored in the ways that Spirit cares for us and helps us to navigate our lives on Earth.

In the physical world around us and in all the social morality that has grown out of our physical existence, there are rules and choices that govern what we can and cannot do. Here we notice that the laws of duality are in charge: the Yes/No of choice; the Up and Down of scale, Big or Small; the Darkness versus the Light; our Mama for nurture and our Papa for power. As it is in the physical world, so it is with our personal choices. Between the two opposites there are infinite shades of colour, but in essence we are always choosing less or more of this or that.

At the edge of experience where change happens, all possible variables and avenues are open, ready and waiting for us to decide and presenting us with a multitude of choices, each with its double aspect: open / closed, free / imprisoned, comforting / painful, exciting / boring. As we discover, all variables contain positive and uplifting outcomes as well as less desirable possibilities such as loss, pain, agony, anger, sorrow and irritation. Yet each double aspect helps us to decide what we prefer and we are constantly refining our choices. The choices we call "less good" play their part by helping us to decide with greater clarity what we prefer now.

For example, we all hope to gain approval, validation and love from other people. But when our hopes for progress rest with others, or we constantly seek permission to act, we may find ourselves becoming bored, frustrated, or selling ourselves short by not taking enough time to think or care about what we would prefer and honouring our choices. If ignoring or discounting our preferences is deeply ingrained, there will come a time when we may either sink and disappear altogether into the fabric of other people's expectations, or we feel impelled to make changes that cause us to act "out of character".

What appears as unusual behaviour is often the self-certainty that we have been searching for. At times like these, it is the choosing that matters, almost more than the choices. If we have been unused to deciding anything for ourselves, we may find that we make a great many "wrong" decisions, while we are in a steep learning curve. But even our difficult choices serve us, by revealing what we prefer and making the easier, lighter path increasingly self-evident.

If we ignore a prompt – to slow down, take it easy, rest, write a CV, take some long overdue exercise, eat a lovely meal in a leisurely fashion, visit a friend or make time for that telephone call – the advice will not go away, but will probably return in our dreams or when we are in a period of rest, since in that state we are more open to guidance.

All guidance from Spirit is sent to help us, to en-lighten us, keep us safe or in answer to our prayers – for prosperity, for meaning or fulfilment – so why do we resist? If we might stop searching so hard and learn to listen peacefully, the process of waiting for guidance from Spirit is a reliable way to find answers that resonate with our deepest reasons for being here and with our highest purposes. In that process, we cannot help but awaken to the knowledge of our partnership with Spirit.

Just as the Earth must, we also deserve to find the balance and equilibrium that enables us to live flexibly and enjoyably. If we are too solemn, the world will be a darker place than it needs to be; if we are too careless, we may spend many years going round in circles; and if we are frightened to trust, we may get stuck pondering all the different options open to us, instead of choosing and moving forward with clarity.

It has taken me many years to cast off the habits of negative thinking that I developed as a child and refined into a form of personal torture as a young adult. My mind-set seemed to prove to me repeatedly and relentlessly that any attempts at living purposefully were deluded and pointless and that my hopes would forever come to nothing. Free will supported my negative thoughts about myself, frequently in very destructive patterns. These days, I try not to give myself a hard time over how many opportunities I have squandered and how often I sat around feeling hopeless instead of taking chances, taking measured risks and learning from them.

After all, if I had known any better, if I had known what I might do to change the situation, I would hardly have chosen to act as I did. I knew that my coping methods were destructive, but had very little idea that any alternatives were possible. I was closed off and became, over a period of decades, virtually monosyllabic. Unable to speak about my sense of loss, increasingly I listened, turned inward and waited. While that did leave me isolated, it began a process of opening to guidance from Spirit, which has taken years to trust, accept and learn to follow. Thankfully, Spirit never gives up on us.

To help move myself forward, it has been very important to contain negative feelings and learn to look past them, instead of getting pulled back down into the old ways of thinking. Here is one dream that I had, which reminded me so forcefully about the importance of letting go of negative thinking.

A dream about a conference on depression – I am something of an expert. What starts out as a fairly active series of images, slides into a tableau, a warning. I am at a picnic by a lake, with many others. We are enjoying a day out in the open, very Victoriana and posh with picnic hampers, cutlery, linen and ladies in long, elegant dresses. We know that the lower half of the village which is our destination has been utterly destroyed. Only the upper half is still intact. We enact the drama – this is the ego speaking – of heedlessly choosing to follow there for our picnic. Perhaps we think it has nothing to do with us.

Suddenly we are aware that Grandma has been killed by an assassin from behind whom we cannot see. A ghost with a knife intent on our deaths because we killed it! There is a general panic and fleeing, trying to get away. To get up, up the hill – out of the depression! – the young girls put on their aquamarine silk dresses and flee in a para-lyzed panic. We are not going anywhere fast enough. A revenge killer is claiming the lives of those on the other side of the lake though some do manage to get away… Do I? I cannot recall. My body is frozen with anxiety and I cannot get up onto my horse to escape but maybe they do not reach me. Whoever they are, they are unseen and deadly.

I woke up from this filled with a sense of urgency. Scared and at a loss, I quickly wrote down what I remembered. Later that day I went back to read and ponder. I felt this message was telling me forcefully that I must stay away from the depths of introspection and feelings of unhappiness. They are harmful and careless wallowing would be costly to me – no picnic. I must be more careful of the feelings and sentiments I allow myself to swim around in. When negativity takes a hold, I must divert it to something harmless or offer it up to the angels for my own protection.

Another dream of being in the Indian jungle – foreign territory – and I glimpse at my feet an enormous crocodile with big eyes and large teeth. Like in the Roald Dahl story, this croc was lurking in the long grass – kicking dreams into the long grass? But I could escape easily, by getting up onto the shoulders of the nearby elephant which would save me, lifting and carrying me up higher, nearer the light.

The elephant feels like my husband might, with his strength which he shares with me willingly and which will carry me easily away to safety.

Over many years, dreams have reassured me and subtly changed the way I use my mind and deploy my creative talents. I know now that our beliefs, thoughts and feelings are creative. And listening to dreams – and more importantly, taking the time to learn from them – has reassured me that we are not alone and that Spirit coaxes and encourages us. So long as we can trust, we can join in the dance with other powers of the Universe.

LISTENING LESSONS

I have read a great deal of esoteric Christian literature. It interests me, though I make no claim to study it with great seriousness. Perhaps that is because I am unused to taking myself seriously, or perhaps I am a spiritual tourist. At school I had a girlish crush on Jesus of Nazareth and toyed with the idea of becoming a nun. I have spent much time in the midst of conventional Protestant doctrines, wriggling uncomfortably and longing to be grown up so I could argue and protest. Now I am a member of the Religious Society of Friends in Britain, known as Quakers; and about once a month I venture out to a meeting of Spiritualists where demonstrations of clairvoyance are given, the intention of which is to bring comfort and advice to the audience and in passing, to demonstrate that Spirit lives on after "death".

Spirit take every opportunity to communicate with us, when our minds are quiet, or perhaps while we are engaged in some daily routine that doesn't require much thought, but which helps to turn down the volume of our mind chatter. Then, there is room to drop in hints that help us to join together a few more pieces of the jigsaw.

Working at the kitchen sink recently, I realized that I have a truly excellent reason for not letting anger, sorrow, pain or humiliation rule me: it is far easier to learn the lessons of forgiveness and love while I'm still here on Earth than it would be to wait until I "die", only then to realize the extent of my errors and try desperately to make amends for all the upset and misery I caused while I was Fran Macilvey in a physical body. Seen from that perspective, our failures to accept and forgive are wasted opportunities.

It may be that after "death" we move up to the next dimension, from where we can see how our actions have impacted other people. As well as all the good we achieved, we may be able to see clearly all the pain we caused. What if we are stricken with remorse and expend a lot of energy trying to communicate with those whom we left behind on Earth, to tell them that we understand now how they must have felt and we are sorry that we were not more loving when we had the opportunity? What if these we are trying to reach don't believe in heaven, never go near an optimism circle and don't believe in angels? Might they be deaf to our whispers? Will they ignore the flickering lights and think that the smell of their favourite perfume, by which we hope to attract their attention, is only the smell of carpet shampoo? What then?

We might have to wait until they also die and have joined us before we can finally embrace them and ask for forgiveness, as well as joking, "I told you there was nothing to worry about. Yes, that was me watching over you. Yes, that was me playing with the lights and yes, I know you like the smell of carnations. I was trying to get your attention!"

It was a small but significant realization, as I was standing washing dishes, that there is no need to make my life any more difficult than it already is by behaving badly. I am on a mission. I am going to get my apologies dealt with and my bridges built. I want to make amends now while I can, by picking up the phone, emailing, or sending a letter. What is more, I desire to make my life more of an ongoing miracle by never again allowing deep anger or sorrow to ruin me or leave behind lasting regrets and guilt.

I resolve and intend to build a life filled with light, colour, laughter and joy, all of which is pure self-interest, I assure you: when I die I would like to do so with a fairly clear conscience. The extent to which I fail to forgive myself and others is exactly the extent to which I condemn myself. When God at the pearly gates is looking at my time sheet, I want to be able to smile and say, "Yes, I knew I could do it! And thanks for all your messages and the help you sent. You really supported me by:

~ giving me the friends and family and the hard life lessons I needed in order to learn and make progress in this life;

~ showing me where to go for help and advice;

~ teaching me how to love and listen to you;

~ staying my hand when I wanted to rush off and do the wrong thing;

~ guiding me to read books that would help me;

~ giving me the patience, courage and strength to learn self-respect and to practise my lessons during my lifetime;

~ showing me how to share with others;

~ teaching me the value of forgiveness and letting go;

~ sending me healing dreams to soothe my hurts when I failed to do that for myself;

~ giving me a sense of humour and friends who understand it;

~ keeping my heart strong and my feet facing the right way;

~ answering all my questions with infinite patience;

Whatever I was doing, miracles came to me and showered me with blessings."

When I look back at life, I want to be able to add that I could see miracles surrounding me, offering me reassurance that help was constantly at my side. I would like to notice that I was always blessed, because I was brave and allowed Life to help me navigate the right path.

One cause of the particular depression I experience is that I am accustomed to waiting around for information, approval, permission or the "green light" from other people: from my mother, from my husband, from employers, even from Spirit, whom I have been hoping would *tell me what to do, please...!* When I fall back into the habit of looking for too much strength and support from outside myself, I feel off-balance and uncertain again. I forget that the best and most honest answers can be found when I quieten myself and go within; and that my choices and decisions, even when they may be mistaken, have as much validity as anyone else's. If I am able to act courageously according to my own deepest wishes, who knows how Spirit will support my choices?

I have probably made more independent decisions in the last five years than in the whole of my previous lifetime. For me to decide, and to follow through with a decision and accept the consequences, is still a relative novelty; and many of the difficulties that have arisen have probably been my apprenticeship in decision-making. When we learn to listen, we can become an originator of our changes. When we decide something and are clear about why, when we have the courage to take action, we are setting in train the process where our choices manifest for us. Mistakes are only outcomes that help us to decide what works better so that we are continually moving forward with increasing confidence. Such self-belief feeds miracles every day, as this waking dream sequence shows.

> Follow the seam of happiness! It may be a thin seam of gold, the merest streak in the grey slate, but as you see it and follow it, it will open up for you in unexpected ways. Slate splits, moves and widens out into shining, flexible streams.
>
> God uses experience to tell us what to do. That is one way she especially talks to us, invites us to listen. Therefore, when a project does not work and is repeatedly wrong or frustrating, it is not the right path for us. We are being invited to turn away. To act in accordance with our higher purposes, we turn away from what does not turn us on. To make progress with what matters to us – literally, what becomes matter – we are invited to take the path that welcomes our contribution. Within the satisfaction of our

higher purposes will be our opportunities to serve; and with this schema there is no conflict or worry or doubt or fear or regret. Follow your heart. Listen to your heart. And allow the rest to resolve by some other way. It is obvious – you know! – that to be unhappy is a waste of time, that our contributions are wasted unless given sincerely and happily, joyfully. So go forth and be joyful and step lightly over the paths of others...

LIFE AND DEATH

I like to believe in some form of life after death. More accurately, I believe that there are different levels or dimensions of living. I suspect that we live here on Earth for a while until our physical bodies are cast off at death; that at death, our energy leaves, and goes away to rest somewhere else. We may take on the appearance we had at the time we were happiest on Earth, or we may simply choose an appearance that another person would recognize if and when they happened to find us in their dreams. Later, I believe we may choose to return to Earth in a new body for another life in another place and time.

What our soul chooses to do depends on what it seeks to learn, since, from a higher perspective we all wish to make progress; by which I mean, we look for new ways to grow from the idea of our separate uniqueness back to understanding and unity. When we have reached unity, we may move apart and then, eventually, back to unity again. We are elements within a much larger process of constant change: from movement to stillness, from quietness to action and back. You may ask, why? Well, if we live forever, we need something to do!

While in a physical body, the material distractions of being on Earth serve several purposes. Our five senses help our bodies and minds to stay anchored in the physical world: touch, sight, hearing, smell and taste make the world real to us, and the general hubbub we generate through life helps to anchor us in the reality of this existence; a process which has its uses. When I, for one reason or another, forget to speak to people for any length of time or forget to go out and be part of something active, I can become very spaced out, which is sometimes unhelpful. Not being sufficiently grounded, it can be much harder to contemplate the practical routines that need attending to every day.

Our senses also serve us by making real the illusion that we are separate persons, each existing apart from others and independent. Why would that be useful? Well, it's a bit like knowing what bitter tastes like, so that you can recognise and move towards the sweetness. Too much sweetness and you long for bitter. A life of bitterness and we yearn for the comfort of sweetness. We are constantly moving from an awareness of our separate identity, to a state in which we acknowledge our Unity with Source and away again. In this process, our senses help to maintain the illusion of our separateness, which in its turn helps us to remember the Unity that underpins all our seemingly separate purposes. We cannot be in one state – say, at a point where we recognize our Unity – unless we are able, at the same time, to acknowledge our separateness.

In the awareness that arises from all of our life's choices, we are constantly choosing between one state of being and the other. Like the mixture of hot and cold water, we need an awareness of both, to choose and enjoy either. Ultimately, we move to the understanding that both Unity and Separation can and do co-exist and that each are facets of the other.

Source relishes our happiness and fulfilment and helps us to reach our best potential in every way that we can. When we are working in harmony with our soul's purposes we feel true satisfaction and are energized to meet every challenge on our path with a more peaceful equanimity. We have all come here to make soul progress. Some of us are content to simply experience things. Some of us are happiest when we are learning. Most of us choose to come here because the atmosphere of the blue planet is excellent for the release of negativity and for learning lessons that allow our soul to progress.

The value of life becomes increasingly apparent when we live it to the best of our ability with what we have. Increasingly, Life becomes an endless series of opportunities to prove to ourselves how much we can achieve, which sounds easy – but it's not. Along with our inherent beauty and talents, we bring into this life an assortment of personal traits, preferences and certain weaknesses that can, if we let them, make our lives challenging and unnecessarily difficult. A tendency to be introspective, say, or an addictive streak, might need to be carefully managed. We may have chosen these weaknesses to work on so that we might grow stronger in overcoming them. If we fail in the attempt, we may have to come back again and face the same lessons.

Our most useful lessons are often the hardest and most painful; and though some aspects of our earthly character may seem to make our lives well-nigh impossible, our soul may have chosen to work with and through certain personality traits which we have chosen – in between lives, as part of Soul – to help us to make spiritual progress. Our souls may have chosen to learn difficult lessons during this lifetime; and the progress or evolution of both our "small" soul and the larger "collective" Soul is meaningful.

There is no guarantee that a personality and a soul will have the same complexion or always work in agreement with one another. Perhaps a personality is contrary, demanding and prone to unhappiness. It may have been invested with these qualities because learning to handle such characteristics effectively is one way to discover the value of compassion and empathy. It makes for a harder life, but a quicker lesson: as with all difficult lessons, there comes a time when these will have been learned. When we finally recognize that the purpose of acquiring patience, tolerance, generosity and peacefulness, is to make *our* lives more enjoyable, our lives become increasingly fulfilling.

Whatever challenges we face, we are invited to ask for help with every step of our journey. And when we allow ourselves time for this, every challenge we meet becomes an opportunity. So, feeling playful and following advice offered in the Abraham/Hicks books (6) I have been sending all my concerns off to "My Chief Executive" who is the person in my employ – the guy in the sky – who looks after my life and sorts everything out. In an early morning conversation, it was suggested with a chuckle that I call my employee Davie and think of him as the Universal Organizer. That makes us a Duo, a team working together to make miracles. Knowing that I am not alone when I have to decide has been such a precious, liberating discovery.

Perhaps "God the Parent" knows everything; and in order to know what that feels like, s/he sends her children to Earth for experiences. For the fullest experiences, both the knower and the experiencer work together as a team. Together in their most abundant expression, they realize between them a third aspect, which is simply Being: being together in love feels like a wonderful place to pause the journey, or to start something new. Nothing truly comes to an end, but moves endlessly in a cycle of renewal.

Like the process of creation which works away quietly within our thoughts, words and deeds, patterns in three aspects feel seamless, circular and endlessly renewing. Patterns of three suggest the nature of creation. Triads include:

~ Life the Parent => Life the Child =>
  Life the Holy Spirit

~ Knowing => Experiencing => Being

~ Thought => Word => Deed

~ To Be => To Do => To Have

~ Past => Present => Future

~ Birth => Life=> Death

~ Breathing in => Breathing Out=> Pausing

Miracles are part of divine patterning, which originates in and with the World of Light, from where Spirit moves. In the World of Spirit there is no past, no future, no time as we understand it. Therefore every aspect of creative work, or miracles if you prefer, happens in the eternal "Now".

Everything that exists on Earth has its first origins in the light and is therefore an essential part of the whole, contributing its own unique and elegant perfection. Coming from the Light, earthing, meshing and appearing to us within the construct we call "Time", each aspect of miracle-making feeds each other part and moves onwards in a seamless, never-ending whole. Endless change and renewal is what we witness when we watch leaves unfurling on trees in early spring, or dropping to the ground in autumn, or branches hanging bare in the cold breezes of winter as their roots rest underground. The cycle never ends but goes on beyond what we can see, continuing into infinity.

For many weeks I have been pondering the Chariot Wheel symbol. It is all in one golden piece, representing endless movement, just as Karma is. Karma is the Sanskrit word for wheel. I best render its likeness in golden chalk, softening the outlines. The wheel of light cannot be delineated exactly. Lines are not in its nature.

The contrast between the light of the wheel and the shadows between the struts, became the idea that earthly life is more like a photographic negative than we realize. When we hold old-fashioned photographic negatives up to the light, we see the bulk of people's heaviness, or things shown in dark patches. Similarly, if our life on Earth is the negative, the photographic positive must be the realms of light or heaven, where all those heavy blue shapes are filled with brightness.

Our bodies in their higher, brighter reality are more radiant, light filled, with the merest sketch for hands and features, the boundaries of which we call our outline. To breathe in is to take in light-ness, to fill our bodies with light, a stream of gold being breathed into the darker, weightier blue which is the heaviness of Earth life.

And later, another understanding along the same lines swam to the surface. A tree takes in light and air; and from the air makes leaves, a trunk and solid, heavy roots. Light and air are fixed in the soil. From its breathing, a tree makes more solidity; makes beautiful soil, muck which fertilizes the tree and allows it to grow ever higher and stronger, to reach for more of the light above. In exactly the same way we reach for light and air by breathing deeply. Thus we bring down light into our lives, anchor it and pull it to us with each breath.

There is great beauty in light and shade, in sublime shadows and loam, all together in one synthesis which is all part of the mesh, the puzzle, the knowing. We are all playing in this together. We incarnate, like trees do, and have the same task as them: to bring light to Earth, to anchor it and display it in beauty. That is why we are all here. And the trees are kindred spirits.

All of incarnate life is here to import light from the world of Spirit! Some, by being darker, show us the light by allowing the play of contrasts to be more obvious. All of life is joined in the great enterprise to lighten, to sweeten, to embrace and display love.

Our eyes can and do notice miracles moving, but we look past them, discount them or ignore them. We call what happens to us a trick of the light or coincidence; we say we don't believe it; we let "luck" drop to one side and walk on by. Perhaps the trick is to accept that a lovely series of seemingly connected occurrences forms part of a message which we can turn to our advantage. We can insinuate ourselves, joining in the dance. When we join with a feeling of relaxed enjoyment, we soon find ourselves moving into other states of awareness without thought.

When I am able to glimpse nature at its wildest, I sometimes feel that I am watching an unfolding miracle. So closely do wild creatures live within their natural environments that it is hard to know where a creature and its environment stand apart. The state of mutual dependence within natural landscapes is so complete – and so complex – that it feeds and maintains itself within a perpetual loop which is continually growing and expanding to enclose every-thing within it.

We take wild animals into captivity because we admire their beauty or singularity and their difference from us. We admire their silken fur, their wild crying, we envy their connection with the planet. We see an-imals or plants as fragile and we bemoan their loss: we think of having or losing, another perception in two halves. But while we obsess about form, shape, colour and texture in isolation, we are unaware that without their natural environments in which they can be themselves, the animals and plants we gaze at behind barbed wire are less than half alive. So keen is their feel for their own habitat that without it, their physical beauty tarnishes. Without the shadows of nature that complement it, feed it and nurture it, allowing it to be itself, the wild wilts and loses much of its meaning and purpose.

The true spirit of wilderness cannot be known in isolation. All its parts together move in glorious pat-terns which make of life a beauty that is more than the sum of each part. That "something" is intangible. Have you noticed how a seashell looks beautiful on a beach, but if you take it home and prop it on a shelf, it soon looks tired and uninteresting? The beauty on a beach is not only about the sand, or the water lifting and falling, or the shells or the crabs, but is what happens when these all are living in the same place at the same time, existing and moving with and for each other. The wild is an essential aspect of who we are too, since it reminds us that we are part of a bigger picture. We catch fleeting glimpses of wider possibilities when we allow ourselves to dream.

We may still insist that we cannot believe anything miraculous ever happens to us. Even as we are standing at the seashore, we insist that miracles are certainly not part of our lives and we don't believe they ever will be, until we have seen their so-called power with our own eyes. Very often I slip into this everyday cynicism, lazily accepting that my time must be spent plodding forward with my eyes cast modestly down. Living by reacting to what "happens to me" is one main reason why I get unhappy and depressed. Living reactively is understandable, yet it leaves me feeling chilled and hopeless.

For a bit of permanent refreshment, I am beginning to turn everything upside down and exercise my power more consciously. What do I choose to do now? Where shall I place my thoughts and beliefs? Even when I am trapped in a myriad of daily jobs that I don't feel I have exactly chosen, how shall I engage with them and colour them in? How shall I see myself working in the world? Is my seashore relaxing and well ordered, or is it a chaotic mess, with detritus washing up around my feet? What I believe is reflected in everything I see.

The outcomes of our thoughts are easiest to notice in our personal relationships: is my spouse interested in what I say, or does s/he pass politely by? Instead of getting cross, can I check, does their behaviour reflect mine? Am I distant and unavailable? When I ask my daughter what she has been doing at school she answers "stuff". Is this because she is naturally bored with me? Or is she disinterested because I rarely listen to her? If I deliberately make time to listen when she comes home from school, how might the conversation turn out differently?

When I believe that I can influence things for the better, I watch for the difference my thoughts and decisions make. More usually, we act unthinkingly and enter the arena at the second stage: we see what we expect to see, little realizing the role our expectations have played in the creation of what we see.

If we are creators, then everything we feel, think, say and do has consequences. We are always poised at the cutting edge of our own creating. If we are creators first, we smile. We can be in at the start. As we express the power within us, it gathers strength and conviction and we can see all the ways in which our thoughts, our ideas and our hopes shape our lives.

WHAT MATTERS TO YOU?

For many of us, miracles remain tied to a magic that procures something out of nothing: the miracle of the loaves and fishes; Jesus bringing Lazarus back to life; the wedding feast at Canna where the wine never ran out; the curing of leprosy and blindness.

In the beginning was The Word; and The Word was God / Life / Love / Source / All That Is. Knowledge common to all spiritual traditions is that Mind came first and made the body; which means that as we think about things and offer them our energy and focus, they are drawn towards us. What we believe then becomes true for us.

If we take a look at our language, we will find clues that remind us of this. For example, the title of my book *Happiness Matters* is fortuitous. Because happiness is a state of joy for what is, happiness

– produces that state where our ability to manifest what makes us joyful becomes a skill we increasingly take for granted;

– is in itself an acknowledgement that the outcome we enjoy is already here. We are already happy; therefore

– happiness – and joy, peace, serenity...positive states of being are the source of all fulfilment and its best reward. Uplifting states of being are both fulfilment and the source of fulfilment.

When we can be joyful – in whatever way we can make that happen! – we discover that we do things because we are filled with joy. In that state, what we desire is drawn towards us and feeds our positive state all the more.

It is hard for us to realise that at some level, we are always choosing everything we think, say and do. It is even more challenging to accept that our choices literally matter. They make the difference. We own them = we speak about them = we admit them = we give them admission. When we say that a thing "matters" to us, our creative drive about that thing absorbs our energy and so we are already bringing that matter into being. If something matters, we think it is important to us. If we import something = we bring it to us from elsewhere = it comes to us = we make it important = it matters = it materializes for us.

Words and phrases scattered through our lexicon reflect a truth back to us, that what we *think* is import-ant and comes to us as stuff. We cannot summon what we desire with the *body,* though naturally our bodies house the *animus* which allows us our fullest expression. In response to prompts from our sixth sense, our intuition, our hunches…we are always summoning with our energies (spirit) what we expect or hope for. And very gradually, our awareness is vindicated that our spirits lead and enlighten as the body follows. Of course, without our bodies, nothing can be manifest, and in any case, the body is very largely made up of air, light, and intangibles which are akin to spirit.

And in the midst of all our creating, the Universe makes no judgement but watches what we do with our power. Miracles take this natural process of creation a step further, arising as they often do from our realisation of our power, supported by an awareness that what we desire is already with us. (Since time does not exist, all must exist in the constant present.)

Just as we cannot summon what we desire with the body, making demands through gritted teeth is unlikely to be fruitful. Our willingness to apply ourselves to our choices takes us a long way, since our commitment helps consolidate our desire and focus our intention. We need to prove that we mean what we intend, and for that, a bit of effort is crucial to help us decide what matters. But it is easier to work productively if we can set aside our belief that work is a constant, uphill struggle. Any attitude akin to pushing, shoving, worrying, endless calculation or comparison reeks of doubt and throws difficulties and upset into the unfolding path of any outcomes.

We all have access to soul wisdom and energy to bring more hope into our lives. Spirit recently sent me a picture of a coal delivery, new coals over the old, until my coal bunker was overflowing, signifying new help and strength coming to help stoke the fire of my focus.

As well as asking directly for help with particular issues, we can work with dream pictures quite consciously to move past a problem or question we may have (as I did with that somersaulting tree).

Think of any situation that preoccupies you or makes you unhappy. Closing your eyes, take a snapshot of that matter and bring it into focus. Study it as a photographer would, with a calculating eye, considering perspective and shadow. Observe it. See it, but know that it is better for you if you suspend all feelings and judgements. As you observe, release emotions, to help you see it clearly. Once you have a picture, you can do many things with it; for example you might:

~ Watch it shrinking until it is the size of a postage stamp. Stick it on a letter and see yourself posting it away.

~ Bleach the colour out of it, until it fades, crumbles and is blown away like the scraps of a pale autumn leaf.

~ Fold your photograph into the shape of a toy boat which dissolves on contact with water and disappears.

As well as casting off a difficult situation to bring in healing, take the opportunity to ask for and invite in any new pictures, as many happy solutions as you like. As you invite them, they come to you. Now, you may put as much emotion, feeling and desire into your *solutions* as you like. Pour real joy and laughter into these. Dream up the solutions you would like to see, so that perhaps:

~ Your boss comes over to your desk and offers you a heartfelt apology for all the unpaid overtime you put in, as well as a pay rise and a couple of weeks' holiday.

~ Your colleague apologizes for being rude and invites you out for lunch.

~ Your mother phones you after the kids are in bed and you have something wonderful to tell her. She listens kindly and you laugh together. In what you talk about, you hear that she is very proud of what you have achieved, and with your shared joy and understanding, you bless each other.

~ You and your partner make love all afternoon while the neighbours' children invite your children over to join their games.

~ All the help you need comes to you from an unexpected source, allowing you to have a restful and fulfilling day.

When miracles are at work, everyone wins.

To set the ball rolling, it is easier to ask sincerely, then follow promptings and put in the hard work as and when we are led to a purpose. If we make our sincere request and then effectively forget about it – while we do something enjoyable which raises our energy – the Universe is working away in the background, figuring out a way to bring us what we desire. We can assist that process by releasing doubts. We have nothing to lose by trusting guidance and living in faith. Cheerful waiting is always helpful, whereas worries are paralyzing.

Though the intensity of our desire does create a strong current towards fulfilment, it helps the outcome if, when we are clear about what we choose, we can relax and let go of our usual anxious oversight. To forget that we made a request is better than remembering we do not have our answer yet. Since it is hard for us to wait for our prayers to be answered without becoming disheartened, Life secures a happier outcome if we make a request and then get busy with something else. Here, forgetfulness is the way, so long as in the meantime we do something – anything – which refreshes and uplifts us while we wait.

JESHUA OF NAZARETH

The dichotomy that traditional church teachings offer of the life and teachings of Jesus of Nazareth has always intrigued me. Even as a young child I understood that Jesus was gentleness and supreme love. So where did hell, sorrow, pain, suffering, guilt and penitence fit in with his messages? I was puzzled. At the heart of traditional Christian doctrine there seems to be a problem: if the established churches practiced what Jesus preached, they would scarcely exist.

So the picture we have been bequeathed by the Establishment is of a Jesus fuzzy around the edges, emasculated instead of powerful, although some of the messages he gave are very threatening to the established order: "Again I tell you, it is easier for a camel to go through the eye of a needle than for someone who is rich to enter the kingdom of God." (7) Not much comfort there for the wealthy.

I have always wanted to understand the real Jesus. I hope you will not consider me presumptuous if I include the following sequences which are the result of my seeking. It is not my intention to question or discount the value of your personal beliefs and experiences, but to show, if I may, how far an ordinary person can walk with revelation. Through the years I have asked for help and guidance and these dream sequences have come to me. In some way, we can each receive personal guidance which is powerful and transformative, as this has been for me.

Jeshua of Nazareth was a prophet. A man like men and so, like us. Either he is the son of God – and so are we – or he is not and we are like him in this way. His whole message was that he is the same as us; that if we follow his example, we can find ourselves as powerfully as he did. That is what he came to preach and with God's help, this is what he came to show us. Our true natures are part of Spirit, filled with light. That is what he was trying to tell us: that our bodies are for a time in the heavy – dark – atmosphere of Earth, wherein we can import love – light – with our acts of peace and joy. By being joyful and honouring our divine light, we bring the light of Heaven to Earth. This is the parting of the veil, the thin blue line separating our "real" world from the place of light, whence all children come.

Perhaps our actions can be read inversed also: that giving is better than receiving, that our greatest misfortunes in this life may be counted as some of our greatest triumphs in the light world...

Pieces of the jigsaw were fitting together so fast it was making my head spin:

Jesus did not come to Earth to "suffer and die for our sins". This is the ego spin on a larger mystery that the ego no longer understands nor wishes to understand. Jesus came to Earth not to suffer and die, but to demonstrate that he did not suffer – he was a master in the control of matter with the mind, including his own pain – and that he did not die!

Christians say they believe in eternal life. And Christ is reported to have said (I paraphrase), "All that I have done, you shall do also. Yet, if you cannot believe that of yourselves, then you can believe it of me. See what I have done! – follow me." We may follow his example, if by doing so we find life easier. That is what he meant.

Some weeks after the above sequence came to me, in the early morning I collected this next understanding. Despite the cold and the temptation of my warm bed, I sat up at my desk at 3 a.m. and scribbled as fast as I could, my thoughts spinning:

> What I mean to write is hard to explain, though I shall try. If we live in the present, we cannot be unhappy, since unhappiness is the context of what has been or what will be. Unhappiness has as its seed and fodder the story of our lives. Therefore, the more closely we live in and with the Perfect Present, the harder it is to maintain the unhappiness which lies in what has been or what will be, like a chain.
>
> In other words, God is not so much a story as a state of presence. Like a shaft of light upon the land, God IS; and in the presence of GOD IS LOVE there is nothing to be unhappy about. It is a state of enlightenment, to live in the light, as it passes over the landscape. To step neither to left nor right of it, nor before or behind. Straying behind or ahead means we once again live in the shadow, however slight, of a context, within which context an awareness of unhappiness or sorrow carries itself.

The trick or challenge comes in staying within that narrow band of light which can be called the eternal present – *gift* – the great I AM. The golden shaft of light which falls to Earth and illuminates our being has no past, no future. It IS NOW. And living within that thin band of light we arrive, without thought, planning or endeavour at a state we can call Grace.

Understand that all of Heaven is like this: eternal, peaceful, moving present, without past or future. The great, loving, final, peaceful, patient I AM. Stay with me, it beams at us and says. It makes no promises, yet is infinitely consoling. Stay with me, it says and in my peace all is well. The transcendent state of grace, Nirvana. And it is so easy to "get there". Just be there, now, always. Like the meditation on matter, this conveys the understanding that light is limitless. The present is all one with any past or future.

As if that were not enough, I gain more understanding of The Beatitudes, ("Blessed are the meek" etc.) which seem now to reflect a spiritual understanding that contrary to popular belief, the real world IS the world of light, where we all came from and where we shall all return. In a state of enlightenment, wealth is meaningless and earthly power is equivalent to poverty of expectation. Since all earthly gains cast a shadow, the blessed ARE the poor, the meek, the loving; since the "enlightened" live lightly by living in the present, they are indeed among the blessed. The poor, the meek, they have less baggage. They have fewer trappings and are therefore blessed because their lives do not trap them. They live and travel light.

CHANGING UP A GEAR — EXPONENTIAL POWER

This chapter may send you into an argumentative frenzy, but I invite you to pause and reflect. In the big wide world where miracles are waiting patiently for us to rediscover them, the law of straight lines and predictable, logical outcomes has no hold. Exponentials rule.

What is an exponential? Well, a child at school learns two plus two = four, four plus four = eight and so on. Within the frameworks of reasoning which we call mathematics, arithmetic and logic, these sums hold true. The reasoning we are taught is designed to be predictable, to follow patterns which can be replicated reliably a million times over. Much of our lives are predicated on the assumption that everything can be sorted out reliably, if we simply apply enough logic to a situation. This kind of thinking works well enough within a construct where we can compute all or most of the relevant factors. The urban landscape is a rather good example of one in which most of the relevant variables can be computed in the final result, to produce a predictable outcome. However, it seems to me that these methods contain a flaw, which is the suggestion that for every problem there is a solution with a beginning, a middle and an end; and indeed that there is such a thing as an "end".

In nature there are no ends because if anything ended, Life would eventually be capable of being entirely understood. To understand something completely – to be aware of all the variables in any puzzle – is to come to the finish of it; and in nature, nothing is ever finished. We do not come to the edge of the world and tumble off it, as the medieval mind-set would have had us believe. The world is a sphere, around which we can move for eternity, if we wish. Endings imply a stopping, a death or lack of movement; but life, as we know, is forever moving and changing. Even the pause between the in-breath and the out-breath is merely a state of subdued movement before something more obvious happens.

If we wish to understand nature more sympa-thetically, perhaps we can begin by considering that exponentials are nature's way. An exponential says, "Two plus two = five; five plus five = possibly thirteen; thirteen plus thirteen is somewhere around thir-ty-nine…" With this kind of graph, our sums are very soon off the scale, since an exponential calculation never follows a straight line: straight lines would signal the end of the world, which is something that Life will never allow. Nature has its own agenda, which – no matter how hard we try – we cannot know or understand completely. The only thing about exponential patterns that we can know with any certainty is that they are unpredictable. How scary is that?

Not knowing is so frightening for most of us that we run for cover while trying to remember our sums, as we scratch our heads and mutter incredulously, "Surely this cannot be right, there must be some mistake…" Before long a team of researchers sets up a very detailed experiment, starts an avalanche or whatever, and discovers that, like a tidal wave, all the data comes rushing in at far greater speeds and at far greater depths and heights and widths and all the rest, than *any of us could have predicted.*

If you ponder the rate at which Earth's icebergs and polar icecaps are melting, I suggest that there are only two factors about which we can be certain: that the rate of melt is exponential; and that we do not have and never will have all the "relevant data" we would need to predict rates of melt with any accuracy. The number of variables which affect the outcome and the way they work together is infinite. Not only that, but we can never see the edges of the bigger picture. We have no way of knowing how long we might be safe from rising sea waters or plummeting temperatures, for example. The predictable conclusion is that our forecasts are probably wildly inaccurate. None of which is very reassuring, but then, natural patterns do not exist to provide us with reassurance, but to ensure their own continuation.

Losses in nature happen so quietly that they pass unnoticed until their accumulated effects become too obvious to ignore, at which point it can be too late for us to remedy the situation. We tend to see things happening in isolation: the loss of fish stocks, the melting icecaps, the loss of bees, the effects of deforestation. It is only when we see the results of these losses working together that we realize their cumulative results are far greater than they first appeared to be.

What does any of this have to do with making miracles? Well, looking on the bright side, exponentials remind us that we too are a vital part of nature's limitless patterns. Our bodies contain water, carbon, phosphorous, iron…but we do not know the magical mix that brings them to life. In this sense, we understand that we are far more than the sum of our observable parts.

Our intangible, spiritual aspects relentlessly move us forward, taking us beyond our usual boundaries and limited awareness. Life itself is a process of becoming more than the sum of our parts. If, in choosing what we shall do each day, we can glimpse the way our choices move ahead of us and unfold in patterns we could never have predicted, we are well on our way to understanding how miracles work. We are well on the way to understanding the power of our beliefs about ourselves, as we begin to exercise our faith and know at last that believing is seeing.

In living our lives as well as we can, happiness is more likely to remain with us when we are aware that we are always creating something greater than $1 + 1 = 2$. Becoming conscious of how our power works does feel miraculous. Accepting our personal strength to move and shape our presents and our futures, we cannot help stepping a little farther into our power. We are constantly becoming more, moving beyond, changing what we know and growing in awareness, in exactly the same way as exponentials are. We cannot stop our power from moving us constantly, urging us to become more. If this makes our lives unpredictable, it's a good thing. How does it feel to know that everything is constantly changing and we have limitless choices?

HEALING LIGHT

Dreams that speak to us of our quiet miracles are tailored exactly to what we believe and to our present needs. Belief has come to me after I have regretted being lazy or complacent with the gifts I have received or when I know that I have failed to make the most of my opportunities. Healing dreams can reassure, or less obviously, they can be the wake-up call we need to jolt us into taking a fresh look at our lives.

I asked the angels to heal my concerns. None of these is big, but I know that they puncture my body shield and cause injury. In my dream I was sitting at my desk, where I found gold and silver shields which allow healing to start. Seven colours came to me: from top to bottom, gold, silver, blue, green-blue, yellow, orange and red. I was aware of them within me, in layers, yellow over here, a silver spot there and so forth. Where I needed a colour, there it rested. And then, after I had placed them, they shifted and moved together of their own accord in a brilliant cascade.

I was given to understand that our colours are continuously moving and injury at this level happens when there is lack of movement. The natural order is always for movement. Nothing is fixed, static or stale – all is movement and change. If we can glimpse this even for a moment, we can understand that unhappiness and unease, all boredom, depression and dis-satisfaction come from lack of movement. Obstacles build up, for example, from chronic resentment, which if not moved or washed away, can lead to dis-ease.

This sequence followed some time later.

Useful pictures last night – the first was about colours – considering: in shades from dark to light, which colours are in your body? Where are they placed? Is lots of one colour concentrated in one place, or a little here and there? Some colours will dominate. Dark brown, where does it seem to be? Dark blue, purple, red ochre, all colours lightening gradually…dark purple, light blue, pinks and oranges, yellow.

This is a great way to be refreshingly honest with myself, though I don't need to talk about it. The state of the colours can reflect the state of our mind and body health. Seeing the body in colour, I can feel my way towards understanding, equilibrium and self-acceptance.

Secondly, a nightmare, coming immediately after. This one is quiet, monochrome and heavy with meaning. The grim contrast with the earlier bright colours makes it more shocking. I am a murderer, a quiet one, who sees much, but only from one perspective. All is dark and grey. I go about putting an end to others' lives almost peacefully. There is no charity in what I am doing. I see things only from my perspective, which is how to kill without discovery. Quietly, unobtrusively, using poison, suffocation, cleverness. Clearing away the evidence into dustbins under the eye of cameras, and presumably, having the occasional conversation with others, I do seemingly obvious and normal things while killing. Sometimes I take the notion into my head. At other times I kill "as a favour" to some situation.

What is so awful is not the killing, which

is mostly about the end of breathing and is not very frightening. It is the sense of being completely closed off from other people. All activity and behaviour is about cleverness, quietness, knowingness and avoiding detection. I am, I think (don't we all!) a clever killer who has checked all the angles and done all the considered things. That is frightening, since I can never be honest or spontaneous or say what is on my mind. I am totally isolated from other people and live a dark, haunted and numb existence. Horrible.

I become aware in the final frame that campus is covered in CCTV on the screens of which I am everywhere seen doing seemingly ordinary things with flip top bins, such as wrapping knives in hand towels and casually disposing of them in the ladies' toilet. Such things could, I suppose, be explained away. But there is also, I see it now at last, The All-Seeing Eye from which nothing is hidden and in which all is understood. The Eye does not judge but it knows all: the eye of God. So I have not escaped! Of course not! I should have realized this all along. In fact, we all do know it, but we forget. All is seen and understood.

I wake up suddenly, sweating and filled

with dread. I write these sequences down and ponder their messages for me.

Apart from the obvious understanding that secretiveness cannot hide anything, I know that God would like me to have more fun. And this is because in this life, I CAN have fun! So often before now, I have been unable to enjoy myself because I was focused on achieving something, on being taken seriously, on being understood or searching for answers. But now I have reached a stage where I can have fun and I could make the most of my freedom! Unlike the murderer whose every action is calculated and filled with fear, I am not paralyzed by what I am. Therefore, in gratitude for my freedom I could be happy. I CAN be happy, therefore I should be happy.

The contrast that the nightmare offered with the dream that came immediately before it, underlined a vital understanding: we have a choice between living with full-on colour; or with the flat, grey and isolating loneliness that comes from being too careful, too quiet and filled with dread; which is what my life could become if I do not deliberately choose happiness. Arriving so soon after the colour sequences, the contrast shocked me into an appreciation for spontaneity, for joy and for allowing myself to feel happiness. I know now that being happy is a privilege. Because of the way things are set for me, I can be happy, therefore cheerful openness would be most beneficial for me, as it is for us all, physically, emotionally and spiritually.

Light and colour are inherent in our being and many people can see auras, outlines of energy and light that move around and within our bodies and around natural structures and buildings. If you would like to experiment with different colours to inform and direct your energy, here are a few suggestions. As soon as we begin, we evolve our own understandings:

Green for healing of body, mind, spirit, strength or situations – Everywhere there is any green, healing energies are at work. See trees, grass, leaves flourishing. Where there is **anger or sadness**, use deeper greens to stand firm and regroup. Invite in lighter, brighter, emerald green for refreshment. We can use green to collect volatile red and orange energies from the head and chest – where they may be sitting too high and show up as anger – and channel them down the body to the base. Visualize the body as a tree with deep roots collecting the red and rooting it safely. Red and darker energies from anger, fear or resentment are channelled down into the roots, transmuted harmlessly into browns; and safely anchored at the base, earthed firmly where they can empower and energize without harming. Lighter green foliage unfurls higher up for softer energies, for refreshment and renewal.

Blue for Peace – Earth is the blue planet, bathed in blue, from the seas below and the skies above. The blue of sea and sky, along with the green of natural foliage and tree cover, are Earth's natural cooling systems. Sky and sea support and perpetuate each other, upholding the belt of healing green that supports life. Blue is peaceful, cooling, clearing and calming. Too dark and it veers into depression and isolation; too light and it floats away into sunshine. For intention to calm, wrap sea blues, clear sky blue and azure around you.

Pink for love – see the heart and chest expand with a gentle pink light; light pink expands love. Whichever shade we desire most, we feel it and invite it in, to plug emptiness or loneliness in our heart. We can wrap ourselves up in a pink blanket to soothe, relax and be peaceful. We can call on this pink blanket any time, to soften all our understandings so that others are released from old judgements and allowed to be themselves.

Orange for wholeness and warmth – if you feel chilly or depleted, tired or discouraged, a soothing, smooth orange glow is amazing for repairing and replenishing energy. Whatever depth of orange you need, will come to you with a simple invitation, and you can keep that for as long as you wish. See the glow spreading around you and your situation, restoring it to peaceful equilibrium. As you progress with this, accept any other colours that move in, and allow them to blend and flow.

Red for grounding strength and courage – red, a good pure red, strong and vibrant, replenishes our vital, core energy. We need this, for strength to handle our challenges every day. It will best appear low in our core, at our root, where its power supports and fuels our other energy. If it flares or becomes too hot, or aggressive, calm it with deep purple or green, or visualise it being drawn down, through the soles of your feet, into the earth where it can be put to good use replenishing earth energy, or dissipate harmlessly. If dark red becomes sullen and resentful, lighten it with any other colour, or white to offer the full spectrum of possibility.

Violet for protection – there is nothing to fear. When we are fearful, we can invite and walk in a flame of violet protection which allows in all our good but deflects negative energies and harmful attention from us. While protecting us against hostility and attack, the violet flame burns off any fear we carry within us. We can wrap ourselves in a deep purple cloak of light when we are in unfamiliar or frightening places or situations.

Gold for wisdom – for the Karma wheel, for pain and peace both in their proper place and time. We need challenges, which offer us the gifts of learning, insight, growth, power, strength and renewal. We need time to rest and reflect. The wisdom is to know when to act and when to release. If we desire insight, or peace to be ourselves, we can ask for the gold light of wisdom to come into our bodies and replenish our souls and their purposes for us in this life. The Golden Rule reflects the wisdom of ages and reminds us that it is in our best interests to treat our neighbours as we would like them to treat us. It is wise if we do so, for in the greater scheme of Life our actions return to us, both our unkindness and our generosity of spirit. Gold light is everywhere. We can remember to ask for more gold wisdom when we are making decisions.

White light for any situation – when we feel unsure or unable to help ourselves out of sadness, tiredness, anger or worry; when we do not know what help to offer others; when we are unsure whether help will be welcome, we can wrap ourselves in white light and/ or send a shield of white light to others. Everyone benefits, whatever the situation, and we do not need to know any details.

As a gesture of caring and love, I enjoy asking Spirit to send universal white light to many people and situations and to bring me more white light. Since all colours of the spectrum are held within the white, the person, body or situation I am thinking of receives total energy and can select from it whichever colours or frequencies it prefers. Thus, there is no intrusion, only a gift of power and energy, sent with love and intention to assist in renewal. Light we send out with love acts as a natural catalyst for physical, emotional and spiritual healing. It can be the spark that starts a healing fire.

Colours and shapes pulse with life. Having invited the process, I watch, absorb and listen and have occasionally found myself being carried away on the wave of energy offered in prayers of healing for others. Energy in shimmering colours may move and dance to its own rhythm, taking light and healing where it is most needed, vibrant patterns reaching out to the person for whom the energy is intended. Wherever love moves – and it moves everywhere – there is peace and joy for the taking and the growing knowledge that we are never alone.

Look out for signs that your requests have been heard and are being granted. Does it seem to you that the sun is shining more brightly? Are you suddenly aware of purple flowers? Do you have the urge to go out into a green space? Do you suddenly feel like clearing out your wardrobe or watering your houseplants? Has a butterfly come into the house?

Consider which colours you may wish to hold around yourself for a few hours to strengthen, delight and renew. All this can be done silently with a simple invitation.

Use your time to bless others, to ask for their healing and strength. All the prayers, requests and blessings that we send out for others come back to us multiplied many times over.

THE BIGGER PICTURE

As we begin to learn about miracles, small miraculous happenings become an accepted and welcome part of our lives. Tuned in to appreciate help, we can see the workings of miracles everywhere. Yet, the fact that we can calmly experience coincidences and amazing outcomes in our lives should not lead us to expect that everything will always work out as we think we would like it to.

We are soul in a body, sent to Earth to experience and learn from varying life lessons. Most of the time, we see only a small part of what is happening: one aspect, a few angles, perhaps a couple of perspectives from among thousands. Occasionally we may glimpse a purpose or deeper meaning, but it is rare that total knowledge comes to us. We are not even given complete recall of wonderful dreams which are sent to remind us of our higher purposes. This is another reason why keeping a long-term diary is so precious: we forget; and besides, Spirit cannot send us knowledge of "everything". For everything we cannot understand, there is probably a good reason.

Perhaps we are struggling to come to terms with a challenging relationship and we have to keep working it out, plodding along because Spirit are silent and don't appear to be listening to our requests for help. Perhaps the timing for our various hopes is not right. Revealing meaning might be premature. There may be other things we would benefit from doing and learning about first, experiences we need to go through, before we are ready to understand and profit fully from whatever comes next.

When faced with apparent setbacks, we may be forced to slow down or reconsider. Perhaps we are being given opportunities to discern that a setback is a gift in disguise which allows us to look at a situation differently, eventually yielding new insights. We grow because we are challenged. Our lives are immeasurably richer when we can look apparent adversity in the face and shrug it off with a smile.

Why did I have to wait until I was in my thirties to meet the love of my life? Perhaps if I had met him after leaving school, I would have ignored him. Hardships that came to me in the in-between years have undoubtedly made me a gentler, more accepting woman, more tolerant of others and more appreciative of gentle men in particular.

Nothing that Spirit or our guides show us is intended to tell us what to do, or to dictate our actions or the course of our lives – except in a genuine emergency, when the message will be crystal clear! Revealing too many detailed outcomes prematurely would suggest, firstly, that everything will be plain sailing from now on and we no longer have a lot to do; and secondly, that the end result is fixed. Neither of these assumptions is correct. Our every mood, every moment of each day, makes this or that direction more or less likely. Spirit are glad to offer help whenever we ask for it, while preserving our right to choose, even if our choice is to do nothing. Spirit do not dictate outcomes, however much they are happy to offer encouragement and energy to help us keep going.

We may be sent prompts that now would be a good time to begin a project that we have long held dear, or urgent warnings when we have strayed too far from our chosen path, but in every case, advice and warnings are there as a guide. That all of these hints are for our benefit is obvious, though if you are like me, you may have spent a lifetime being wary and reluctant to move. Until we understand that all advice is solely intended to make our lives easier and more fun, we may be unwilling to listen and stubbornly cling to the notion that we have to do things our way, the hard way, or not at all. We forget how much Spirit love us and that their purpose is to help make our lives more meaningful and enjoyable.

Though we forget why we are here and what our purpose is, we are all important to Life. We spend years looking for meaning and direction in the wrong places and become frustrated and depressed when we cannot find it. In part, this may be because we have been educated away from the spiritual awareness and inward listening that would help us to find answers.

One very ordinary night, in my dreams I was invited back to visit where I had come from. I was shown some of the reasons for my state in life, as well as some of the choices I made while I was in spirit, before I took on the body that is Fran Macilvey. In helping me to understand parts of the bigger picture, I was strengthened to embark on the next chapter of my life – to listen and start taking notes so that I could widen my view. It was many years before I began writing seriously, but my diary notes became steadily more important to me. I know that without all the tears, thinking and hard work that have been poured into my three books to date, I would not be alive now. For me, the disciplines of writing have indeed been a life saver.

There are cynics who would say, "Miracles? What miracles? Have you made a sick man well or turned water into wine? Did you cure leprosy or bring a dying woman back to health? Go away and stop talking nonsense." And there are those who would ask,

"Why would such things happen to him and not to me? Why should I have to suffer and put up with all sorts of indignities? I see precious little compassion in that. You are being cruel, writing about miracles and inviting us on a foolish dance around things you don't understand."

Everything I write comes with the caveat that I write from my own experiences; and nowhere am I saying how things *should* be or what anyone else *should* do. I hope to offer ideas about what *might* be. For too many years, I made my life impossible by resisting the many lessons that my experiences brought me; and I railed bitterly against my life circumstances: to be born with a life-long disability that excluded me from doing what I most enjoy; to be forced to confront the demons of my depression and self-hatred before I was consumed by them. Ultimately, if I was not to die an embittered woman, I had to learn how to love life, and everything in it, gently.

Now I can accept my life as it is. I can love my husband and my daughter wholly and peacefully. I can accept that, however much I may despair about the injustices of life, everything is held by an all-encompassing Light, which loves everything and everyone unconditionally and always. How can Life not love us, when we are all part of the same all-encompassing miracle?

Yet, even Jesus would not heal the sick if that was not what their souls would have chosen. Before personality is born into a body, soul decides what lessons it would like to learn in its next life. The personality within a body may spend years living in harmony with these aims or disputing the soul's choices. The soul's aim is to make spiritual progress. Since our soul is in charge of our spiritual journey, it may decide that spirit in a body might gain extra insight from handling a few challenges: not because Life is unkind but because a personality placed in challenging circumstances will have greater opportunities to learn and grow.

The personality faced with difficult life lessons has two choices. It can resent the life it has, fight, plead, despair, hate and bargain with God (all of which I have tried). Eventually, all that hatred and despair makes us ill and we may sicken and even die because this life lark is too damn hard: the hard challenges our souls took on proved too much. If that is so, we may go home and try in another life to learn similar lessons in a different way, always understanding that no progress we make is ever wasted.

Alternatively, if we endure and come out the other side, we may awaken to more awareness of Spirit. With the gift of our lives, our souls have something to show us; and once we accept that our lives are unfolding as part of a bigger process, we can put down the sword and shield we carry. Following our feelings, hunches, guidance, and our enthusiasms, we can begin to trust our leadings, which, if we allow them to, can show us easier ways towards fulfilment, peace and abundance.

Not everyone chooses to be healed when healing is offered. Healing Now is not always on the cards – unfortunately! Healing will come, certainly, but perhaps not quite Now. To answer that painful question *Why?* when confronted by my tiresome frailties, it helps me to accept that I came to Earth to experience my life as it is, because my experience of life is unique; and because in doing so, I have so many opportunities to learn how to overcome feelings of disadvantage. In discovering the strength that we hold within ourselves to make all kinds of choices whatever our situation, we become stronger and hopefully a little wiser, all excellent reasons why we might choose difficult lessons.

Others may desire to come to Earth so that they may discover what sorrow feels like, or to learn compassion and emotional resilience. Some may wish to learn true empathy or to offer their families opportunities to learn the lessons of caring.

It is relatively easy to see that we may choose to learn lessons which arise from seeing beyond perceived physical or emotional difficulties, from accepting help, and through that process learning to create more joy in our lives. It is more challenging to apply these sorts of explanations to our encounters with those who are unkind, selfish, cruel or dangerous. Where is healing when we need it most?

Free will is part of what makes us human, an aspect that allows us to choose to act in certain ways: to be cruel or kind, to be parsimonious or generous. We are all searching for the same things: we all yearn for love, acceptance, peace, joy, for physical, emotional and spiritual fulfilment, though each of us has different ideas about what these mean and how to achieve them. And thus the tapestry of life evolves. If everyone was saintly, patient and giving, how would we learn the importance of taking care of ourselves, or the wisdom of being thoughtful, courageous, or acting with caution? If everyone was constantly content, when would we appreciate the value of striving for success? You cannot very effectively explain to me how to live well. I really have to learn that for myself, perhaps by choosing clumsily at first and in that way, gradually walking more confidently towards what I prefer.

To set the context for choosing and learning, for becoming more than the sum of our parts, there have to be others, there have to be circumstances and places, there has to be behaviour that we consider to be less than ideal. Given my personal weaknesses, I know that in order to treat my family gently, for example, I had to suffer a bit first, so that I could learn more empathy.

My lessons have mostly been doled out carefully in small steps and I have been greatly helped along the way. There has been sharpness, sorrow and lots of pain – much of it self-inflicted – but most of that, I like to think, is being turned around into something good. Even the things I dignify as "tragedies" in my life have taught me a great deal; and when I look back at how they have shaped me and forced me to grow up, I am immensely grateful for their lessons. The school of hard knocks has shown me the pain that comes from choosing wrongly, and my "mistakes" have made me a kinder, more confident woman. Without the pain, I would be uncertain that my choices now are genuine.

The full spectrum of experience includes all the good and the bad, all the sick and the thriving. There is room for them all in God's creation and they all play their part in allowing each of us to choose what we would like to do next, where we would like to go and what our lives are in the process of becoming. Not all people will be healed and not all will choose to be. There are many paths and many cross-roads. I may meet the sick, the sad and broken on the way and then our paths may diverge. We shall bless each other, but we will not all be walking in the same direction. Not yet.

TWO STEPS FORWARD AND ONE STEP BACK?

Progress through life seems to move rather like a dance, two steps forward and one step back, so that my favourite homilies tend to feature perseverance, hope and continuance in the face of discouragement. Learning to trust divine timing and the unfolding processes of life has been one of my biggest challenges.

At a workshop, our tutor for the evening reminded us that gentleness is a virtue which can be expressed as the opposite of criticism or self-abuse. Another good tool is prioritizing. So I can put the two together and notice that it is helpful for me to prioritize gentleness. To get beyond habits that cause me such regret – impatience and anger are top of the list – prioritising gentleness gives me permission to let go of all the judgement and relax the Calvinistic work ethic that constantly insists on pushing me for results, as if I can sweat my way to serenity.

But some part of me has to be careful too, not

to sink into lassitude and defeatism. To find a balance as I totter through life, I have to listen carefully, treading the delicate line between doing too much, and doing nothing at all. It would be very easy for me to sit and watch, admiring life from the sidelines, without really living.

Historically, I have swung from utter passivity to frantic action and back, but this pattern of doing things is not the most helpful for consistent progress. Why have I swung from side to side? Perhaps because I was frightened to move forward. Many of my dreams and prompts have reminded me of the ongoing challenge of staying steady and calm, even though my balance is poor and my energy tends to flare or die suddenly.

> Recently in the dark early morning I received more answers. I still hold a core belief that "Life is Hard". This may be connected to a weakness cantered around the neck –neck problems can signal stubbornness, fear of letting go or inflexibility. Physical balance is rare for me and that lack of stability is probably mirrored in emotional imbalances. Perhaps that has grown up into a fear of making changes, of moving forward, making choices that will bring emotional and spiritual consequences.

A break in light, in continuity and the flow of energy might also explain a feeling of being stuck, unable to move; being easily upset and unbalanced; not seeing projects through to completion and all too familiar feelings of not being properly rooted. I tend to overcompensate, which is tiring and reinforces the belief that Life is a Struggle. The belief becomes the mother of my reality. The challenge is to find balance and still be loving, gentle, forgiving.

Once I am standing calmly with some degree of stillness, then I must have the courage to go forward. In this, there is less to fear than I thought...

I am sent a picture on the nature of concern. Waiting at the edge of a road with fast moving "dangerous" traffic all along it, it is much too hazardous to cross. So I stand and watch; and I can wait forever OR I can take heed of promptings. Exercising faith with intention, in moving to cross the road, a way is cleared for me. A lollipop lady comes out of nowhere and a path across the traffic shows itself, to allow a smiling lady with a line of schoolchildren – and me – to cross. I am like a child. Still learning and on my way to school, I go with the little ones, who need help to cross the road. I am still an infant, where my learning is concerned. I cannot learn future lessons unless I have faith that the path will clear for me… The way forward opens easily and the cars wait patiently.

Another colourful dream of a cartoon. There is a race and cartoon figures are running round on a track. There is a big hole right through my front, but cartoon figures are indestructible and I keep running until I cross the finishing line. No matter what happens, the race will be run. Also may mean – obstacles are unreal, only there to make us laugh, like "Tom and Jerry". Obstacles that appear daunting are not real and I should not take life so seriously.

The world seems to be full of obstacles which could keep me standing still, watching and doing nothing much. But there is nothing to fear in taking the first steps. There is no real danger out there. Obstacles are an illusion placed before us for our learning and growth. There is nothing to fear in taking steps forward. If I act in faith a way will show itself. I know that God rewards our faith with solutions, if I can remember to act in faith and not by sight! Not blindly, but following God-given prompts.

And in taking steps forward, choosing to take chances, opportunities can unfold as part of a natural process of growth.

I see butterflies everywhere. On the cover of this journal, in books I read and in patterns on children's clothes. We were at "Butterfly World" last week and I have been given a set of butterfly notelets as a present. I think of butterflies all the time. A time of change and moving on? Perhaps a cautious reminder that although life may be lifting off, I need to move gently. For all that they may travel great distances, butterflies are fragile and their beautiful wings are easily destroyed. I must not push too hard.

PAST LIVES

I am finally persuaded to include here a chapter about the rather contentious subject of past lives. It is a very personal subject which I have found rather painful to deal with, but ultimately rewarding. If I can offer my experiences as an example of what can be achieved with a journal, an open mind and a bit of time – in my case, about ten years – it is my hope that you may be helped to find some more of your own answers, though I sincerely hope it does not take you as long.

Relentless pursuit of the question "Why?" creates a craving for satisfaction. I am not dogmatic, only insistent; and anything is worth considering if it will help answer that question. So, along with numerology, astrology, angel therapy, light healing, spiritualism and auras, the subject of past lives has come under the spotlight. While not something to worry or obsess about, I wondered whether this might offer me some clues that I could explore to fill in parts of the puzzle. For a year or so I read every book about past life experiences that I could find, until my interest was sated and most of my questions had been answered. The answers may be right or wrong, but when I am exploring, all paths have value. To me, what matters is finding peace, and answers that resonate with my experiences. That is what makes them "right" for me.

Another piece of the puzzle recently floated within reach, one that I noticed because a pattern was forming. Familiar scenarios unwrapped themselves so often, even the dullest wit had to understand that meaning and purpose was waiting to be recognized. The jolt was almost physical. *Hey! Wake up! We need you to see this.* Repeats in circumstances and familiarities that recycle in recurring themes, don't unspool like a flat photograph, they carry feelings and certainties with them...

Here is a short dream entry that has given me much to consider in the several years since I set it down.

Akashic Records

I went through the forest as I was asked to do. At the edge, I took off my shoes and clothes and was invited to leave them there. I put on a flowing dress and my long, thick brown hair was plaited so that it would not get caught up in the branches of the trees.

Then I walked into and through the forest and into a clearing carpeted with leaves. Up to a tree where there was a door. A climb up many spiralling stairs following close to the roots; through a very small door caked with mud and caught, meshed in roots. Overgrown, it was hard to prise the door open. Not physically possible, but when I stopped trying and applied my clear intention, it was very easy.

From there I emerged into a grand library, pale and circular, with white pillars and subdued colouring. There were lots of distant observers working in among the books. I lifted a small volume out of the shelves. It was not what I expected and I double-checked. Yes, it was definitely the right book, very plain, with a dark blue cover and thin pages, like a Bible. I was told it was "The Book of Sufferings" and that it would get bigger as I looked at it; it would feel big.

I opened the book to a lot of blank pages and saw an evening scene at the pyramids of Giza. Men in white clothing, dancing shadows of firelight; and a very dark, beautiful boy, watching from far off. He has been branded a djinn and bad luck. Ostracized from his group, he looks on as they share an evening meal and talk. I flipped through the pages and saw other scenes, though these I did not pause to consider.

In the midst of my everyday reading, I found yet another book on the subject, which suggested that, without the need to visit a trained therapist, relaxation and visualization can offer us a way to visit past-life memories in the comfort of our own homes. Perhaps, I thought, I might give that a try sometime. Always big on the theory, I resisted doing much about it and let the subject drop. One afternoon several weeks later, the house was quiet so I went and lay on my bed and prayed, again not very clearly, but with a bit of hope, maybe. And this is what came.

Following a suggestion in a book I have been reading, I am to imagine myself sitting in front of a covered mirror, the cover slips off and what do I see? Imagine all the details: fabric, room, comfort, etc…

So, I visualized myself sitting in a chair, in front of a huge, wooden cheval mirror, a tall oval. It swings round on side hinges, flips over and over, so that very soon the dream takes off and pulls itself along without me directing it at all. The mirror moves round faster and faster until it is a blur and I am looking through the middle of the space.

There I see the dark, brooding shape of a small man. Rough stone walls, boulders whitewashed. A bare room. A castle? A keep? The mirror slips and spins and in the centre there is recognition. The man steps out of the flip and up to his ladylove. She is tall, thin, pale and rather neglected, with long curling reddish hair; wearing a long white dress – everyday clothing. He thinks he loves, but he is a bully. She rises to hold his hand because she is well-behaved and they swing round in a tired dance which might, long ago, have been a courtship. He flings her down onto a long trestle table and gripping her cheeks of her face in hard fingers, he has his way with her; brusque and unlovely.

She tolerates it and does not really care about the pain because she wants to get pregnant more than anything and it is a long time happening. For that, she will tolerate all else. Now she has a bump, which she is cradling in her hand when the door opens. She is confronted with a laughing matriarch, coarse and unkind. Is she accused of witchery? Why is there a bump now, after so long? The accusation comes. You have a black cat. You make a pet of it, do you not? Talk to it? You are too old now, too old for a child! There is rivalry between them and the wife is fearful of the outcome.

Later, the picture continues. The flame-haired lady ends up foisted in a cage, suspended over a ravine next to the castle. She is not pregnant but has a stomach tumour. Her husband did not protect her from a public trial. Condemned, she is left in the cage, swinging. But she is ill, past caring and has no appetite. Before she dies, she sings a song, loud, over the valley. Her husband hears and weeps. He realizes he could have used his authority to save her. But she is singing that she loves him still and always will love him. Before, she waited silently and accepting. Now, she has finally spoken out in her defence.

Can one recast the end? See a different outcome? He rescues her as she is near death, retrieves her from the abyss, appalled that his people obeyed his cruelty in having her cast out. He could have protected her but he did not. Still, when she dies they are more reconciled.

After this, a series of past life dreams came to me, all of which had as their theme the paramount importance of maintaining respectability, even though the end result was unhappy.

Another Past Life Regression (PLR)

A young woman is going to be married to an older man of her mother's choice. But she loves a boy, younger than her, perhaps twelve to her sixteen. She leaves him and does marry her older husband. She is obedient. Her husband is a spoiled dolt. She does not love him. She ends up taking to drink and is herself finally cast off by her family in disgrace.

Recast (which is played out very vividly) – she says a sad goodbye to her beloved swain, picks a dark red flower like a peony rose and gives it to him as a token of her everlasting love. But she swears she will work hard at her marriage. She will make sure she has a good solid life and is respected, even if she is not happy. She bids her lover to marry well and swears she will not live to disgrace him. She is seen growing into her late forties or fifties; solid, but not happy. Respected but not fulfilled. She kept her promise but died young in her unhappiness. There was honour, but no fulfilment.

Another PLR

A glimpse of a man in Pharisee clothing, very tall and wearing a high black hat – tall for extra authority – and black robes. Obviously an establishment figure. He is standing away to one side, up on the left, away from the crowd, alone. He is condemning to death someone like Jeshua – Jesus – someone who is entirely innocent. He does this almost without a thought, because that is his job. Positioned where he is, he does not have to see faces. First shock – it is my father; second shock – that judge is also me, condemning a man to a painful death. It feels clear to me that I must now learn the lessons of compassion. Crucifixion. Or, am I the man being crucified? In this life I have a nail through my right ankle. These PLRs all happened on the night of first May, Ascension Day.

And later, a very brief and frightening picture of being caught on a piece of wood and unable to move. A cross bar – crucified? I'm being attacked for some reason that I don't understand. I am a young man, stuck.

Strange, creepy parallels that I could never have imagined are coming to me. Yet, they make strange sense and begin to answer some of my questions. I have a nail in my foot, hammered in there when I was about nine, an innocent. Why did that happen to me? Maybe so that, as part of the process of releasing old Karma, I might learn what pain felt like and become more aware of the need for compassion.

I wrote these sequences as soon as they came to me. The archaic language in the notes – words like "ladylove" and "swain" – I would never use. Yet, as with earlier messages that I have received and needed to write down, I did not wait for daylight. I sat up in the early hours of morning scribbling busily, knowing that otherwise I would miss the chance to reflect on these accounts later.

Whether these passages are real or imaginary, or whether they can be explained logically is unimportant: they woke up some recognition in me. The underlying messages felt familiar: I felt and understood the cruelty of the husband, the passivity of his wife, the sorrow of the married woman, the pain of being crucified and the carelessness of the officiating Pharisee. I could have been any of them. That became a lesson in empathy. The next dreams or PLRs offer echoing themes.

Here is a young boy riding with an older attendant by his side, in a group of initiates all wearing white clothes, robes. I am a privileged boy going to an initiation. We are meeting at a tent in a clearing in the forest. I am to end up in a kind of male brotherhood, feeling isolated, unreal and caught by circumstances again: by my birth, my fate, which traps me in a life where I am well cared for and which others may see as fortunate and privileged, but which is not what I would have chosen.

Finally, there is Cassius Numidius, a Roman centurion who was captured in battle and has lived with his captors for many years. To introduce himself, he wakes me up gently, smiles and offers me a rose, and then his story is told. He is about to go off and fight again and would rather be at home. He is making the best of his life and offers me an ironic grin. He is youthful, clean shaven, handsome and well provided for. He is happy enough, well respected and has adopted many of his captors' customs. But again – he is trapped and unfulfilled. He acknowledges with a sad smile that sooner or later, he will die in battle anyway. He has only been postponing the inevitable.

Looking at these images, I have an opportunity to notice a central, recurring theme emerging as a thread common to all these lives, and indeed, in my own life now: entrapment, and what I can do about that.

In deciding which choices to make in life, there is the path of least resistance, which may offer apparent good fortune and material security but conceals personal emptiness and unhappiness, a sort of living death hidden beneath rigid and stifling respectability. Nothing ventured, nothing gained.

Recasts for past lives can be attempted at any time, simply by asking or hoping for a different outcome. To most of the lives I mention, I have now received positive recasts, an incredibly liberating development which was totally unexpected and which, I hope, suggests that my life is now running along more fruitful lines. The recast for the boy riding to a monastic life – which, with the other recasts, I received several years later – has been particularly helpful and vividly drawn. I offer it here, to show that all circumstances, no matter when or how they have been encountered, can be powerfully redrawn.

The boy riding to the monastic life pulls aside his horse from the midst of the procession and approaches the abbot at the head of the line. He asks to speak to the abbot privately and is granted an audience in a nearby wood, while the abbot orders, "Fill up the line here, from the rear, and wait for me!" The boy kneels and explains that he does not want to go to the monastery. He begs for his freedom and prostrates himself for his request. The abbot loves the boy – a favourite – and grants his request, but says, "I cannot be seen to agree, so I shall imprison you here and you can escape." He drives a sharpened wooden stake into the ground next to the boy, pinning down the white robe the boy is wearing, and as he leaves him in the wood, blesses him with an embrace and a kiss. He throws down a small wrap of coins onto the cloth and the boy is left alone. There is a sense of excitement for the boy's opportunity. He escapes on a white horse.

As the recast shows, my new challenge is to accept what my heart is calling me to do, use my courage and choose for myself, thereby risking the displeasure of others. If I follow my heart there are two possible outcomes: I may succeed – and gain the consent and approval of others! – which takes me further on my journey; or I may fail. If I "crash and burn", that may feel preferable to the sheltered existence I permit myself when I take the safe, "respectable" route and do nothing, which begins to feel like a living death. Cassius Numidius also received a recast.

> Cassius Numidius goes to the camp kitchen, approaches the large soup cauldron. (He is caught up for some very minor infraction and sent to the kitchens to do extra duties.) There he hears murmurs and finally persuades his captors that there is trouble coming. Someone is going to be let into the camp. He is asked to go and fetch help, and he promises to come back. He does return and tries his best to get into the camp, but by then it is over-run. He flees and makes a new life for himself with a wife and family.

Nowadays, there is only one question I need to answer: is this new project something I am willing to try for? Shall I take a risk – usually a small, calculated risk – or shall I simply sit quietly at the side? Let's roll the dice and see what happens, shall we? That does feel like a message for me, come to think of it. If I did not take the decision to commit to something and work on it, my material good fortune could easily keep me sitting still, locked in place. I could effectively choose to do nothing with my life and others, looking in from the outside, would see nothing to regret in that. My private losses would easily pass unnoticed.

It is as well to take the risk that carries the chance of success, rather than sitting around being agreeable and going nowhere. I'm sure Cassius would agree.

In any case, it is no good hiding for the rest of my life, in the hope that everything will go away and leave me in peace. It comes as a shock to realize that in order to make personal progress, the lessons we need to learn will be repeated – and repeated – until we finally accept their challenge and face them. It seems that I must follow my desires and carry through my intentions, despite the apparent difficulties that may seem to crowd out the path, or else, who knows when or how they might show up again. Doing all this work now while I am in a place to understand what is happening will make everything much easier and clearer later on.

Writing three books about my life seems to have brought me full circle. To write about my life as it has been (*Trapped*) I had to notice patterns and choices that I wished to change. To explore happiness (*Happiness Matters*) I dug a bit deeper into personal strength and courage; and in attempting to write this book about miracles, I live with the increasing awareness that we have the power to uncover deeper meaning behind the lessons that challenge us every day.

Without the help of my writing, I would not have done any of this work or made any progress. Nor could I have been told all that I needed to hear in one sitting. I would not have listened. But built up over months and years of "coincidence" and parallels, messages and wonderful, sweet timing, the conclusions become so easy to accept. I can smile at my lessons. At last, I am a happy learner.

SPIRIT SPEAKS

To the question, "What should I do?" Spirit answers, "We have told you many times. Smile. Sing when you would rather cry. Laugh when you feel like weeping. Do not let it matter to you. Act not by sight alone, but with faith that the path that speaks to you of your happiness is the right path, regardless of how it may appear to you, or to others. Spirit speaks in so many ways to everybody. Not with speeches or with grand notions, but simply."

Spirit asks, "If you had all the answers, what would be the point of living? Time and again we speak to you and you do not listen. Rest when you tire; eat when you hunger; sleep when you sleep. You say you wish others would listen to you, but do you listen to us? To take on board our gentle instructions for communion with Spirit is the best way forward.

"All your old ways belabour difficulty, stress or tiredness, but that which we tell you is easy. You can smile now. You can breathe easy. Being true to yourself is the start of a better life for you. A better time for you makes goodness for others. Do not be afraid of what will happen, for the truth that evolves, endures as the fraudulent and the infamous fall away to the outside of your life. Do not fear the unknown. It will pass gifts to you if you will welcome it with acceptance, if you will grin instead of fretting. If you will grow tall instead of shrinking away, we will guide the hand and the foot. We give you time and courage and wisdom and strength to do all that we ask of you. You can all be messengers for God's goodness. If you will not be, then who will?"

"Say 'I understand my God' and 'I praise my God'. All is loved, cherished and drawn towards wholeness. This is the irresistible power that others will try to pull away from and deny. But you know the truth: there is never anything to fear. You will always have everything that you need. Rest now and be calm and happy. We are speaking to you all the time. The first thing for you to do is find inner calm and peace. Then you will more easily hear what is said."

Our inner sense of what is right keeps us on track – if we listen – where our gross senses would mislead because we get caught up in the details. Where the path becomes filled with trips, falls and bumps, it is the wrong path. Smoothness and calm signal that we are back on track.

We are allowed to unburden ourselves, stand aside and surrender to guidance; to take the hints that shower all around us. When I fix and acknowledge the intention, it is done. None of this works in the brain zone: thinking is often where our ego gleefully starts a complex argument with no solution, which pushes goodness away. Truth is nearer to the light than we usually notice; and manifestation happens best in the free-floating zone that sees and responds only with love, with the loving impulse that expresses truth. All creatures can, if we live lightly, be guided by the same transcendent impulse towards love.

Soul reminds me constantly that, "*The soul/sole purpose of the body is for the expression of love in the physical world.*" The soul has a single purpose for our bodies, which is that they be used to express love. By expressing love we bring light to Earth and anchor it around us. That is our aim and our soul's purpose in our bodies being here.

Because physical life is often arduous, there are times when we need reassurance. Spirit happily send gentle dreams of peace and restoration.

I have had a beautiful healing dream of a strong, broad tree, short and stocky, with deep firm roots and full of glowing green strength. Green veins of love and light, pulsing chlorophyll power and purpose. I could see a tracery of veins through the trunk, pulsing with Raphael's emerald-green healing. The tree felt active. Humming with life, it vibrated with energy and light. It feels like I am getting the green light. If this is me, it feels wonderful, as if I am moving, humming in the right way. I may be short, but I am growing stronger all the time.

Other help is on hand. This night I have opened up a book currently at my bedside, *Conversations with God* Volume 3 (8) where I read that, with all my thoughts I am creating. The world follows our idea of ourselves. Therefore it helps me when I can make the highest choice and keep the grandest vision of what I intend for myself.

While doing everything possible to feel better and to surrender doubt, my patience is well directed when I endeavour to see the best in myself and in everyone I encounter. Every thought that is not my highest thought is misdirected, as is the energy I give to those thoughts. With patience and faith, in quietness and trust, my highest vision and my grandest – my most loving – intentions coalesce to show good results.

My highest thoughts are that I am happy; I am free; I am fulfilled; I am at peace with myself. My warring parts are finally laying down their weapons so that the internal struggle is lessening. The battle is ending now. There is peace. Any remaining fears can be mopped up in the arms of love. *I am filled with warm love.*

The only love to offer is unconditional love. The golden rule is to love ourselves as much as we love others: to do gently for ourselves as much as we would do for others. If we love ourselves less than perfectly, to that extent our acceptance is clouded by judgement and with any judgement we condemn ourselves and others to needless suffering. Judgement is condemnation, which affects us and those we judge equally.

> I woke up this morning thinking of three aspects: body – mind – spirit. Which is the most basic? Body, then mind, then spirit. But it became confused, mixed up in my head. It resolves as spirit-mind body, which is the same as soul body. Soul is in charge. I don't need to do anything so much as decide, act in faith and let the soul lead.

HOW TO MAKE A MIRACLE

Congratulations! You already made a miracle – you are here – so the job is done. Nothing more to prove, really, except... Perhaps sometimes we get worried, we obsess over the details, we simply *don't* know what to do, or how to get out of a particular mess.

Do you want to know how we can change that? I've got a few ideas which I've put together into a handy "do it yourself" list, so that anytime you feel doubtful, you can take a look, check and see where your radar is pointing, and maybe make some tiny shifts. That's all it takes – lots and lots of tiny shifts. There is nothing arduous about making miracles, though it does take a bit of concentration, discipline, and watchful attention to how we are feeling, right at this moment.

Tip: Feeling good = the way to go. Feeling not so good = please shift until you feel better. Stay in that better feeling, then shift again to feel better still.

First, go get some genuine **refreshment**. Have fun, rest, relax and take a breather. Eat a nutritious meal and enjoy every mouthful. Go for a walk somewhere pleasant.

Allow, then release, all states of negativity: criticism, judgement, guilt, annoyance, self-pity, embarrassment. Not just about one particular set of circumstances. Release negativity about *everything* you can. (Grief is positive, and expressing grief is natural, necessary and healthy, as long as we are not using grief as our excuse to wallow. Express and eventually lay down your grief, for a while.)

Depending on how you are, releasing negativity can take five minutes, or more likely, it will take a while, so I suggest having to hand some paper and a pen, so that you can make lists of all the things you might like to let go of.

This is to be a fun exercise, by the way, not a heavy, stressed or guilt- ridden attempt to exorcise demons. Just let everything drop. If you need more ideas, you might like to read or revisit my earlier book in this series, *Happiness Matters,* which is full of suggestions you can tailor to suit yourself. Be creative.

Refill your space and your whole life with bright, creative light. Feel the joy that comes from being unencumbered by negative feelings you have shrugged off, finally. Feel open and light.

Go within and listen. The place to start looking for answers is within the self. Can we go within, be peaceful and listen for guidance? Our lives are so routinely noisy and cluttered that we forget how much Spirit yearns to speak to us, which can happen as soon as we open up some space and invite Spirit to communicate with us. This happened to me when I started going to my local Quaker Meeting. Having made the space to be open, Spirit didn't waste a moment, and, for several weeks, flooded me with pictures, explanations and insights, including this one, which remains my favourite.

> So I sat down and opposite me was Christ Jesus sitting on floor cushions, dressed in a kaftan and urging me to play a game of cards. Waiting patiently and urging me to it. I felt bad about that. Didn't want to play. To do so felt frivolous and unseemly, a bit of a waste of time. But I picked up my hand of cards and saw three of the most startling brilliance and dazzling colours – bright pink, deep blue and dazzling green; and they were so beautiful that I could scarcely be prevailed to part with them, even in a game

of cards with God. It was hard for me to part with them. And Jesus said, "You see, I have given you a good hand, so play a good game and have fun."

Decide what you would like to do, be, have or achieve. It can be something very small – I would like to find a parking space – or it can be something more ambitious – I would like to love myself totally, now and always. *I would love to* ... and fill in the blanks by thinking about what makes you feel most alive. Which can take time to work out, or again, it may be a knowing that comes to you very quickly.

Ask for what you would like, clearly, calmly and firmly. Be certain about what that is, and make sure that your request is unambiguous. If you say, "I would like to meet my soul mate, the love of my life," and forget to specify a particular gender preference, for example, the Universe will go to work straight away and cause you to meet the love of your life, your soul mate, who could be any gender. So precision is important, but try to resist compiling a shopping list. "She's got to have great tits and loads of girlfriends," sounds like the ego having a laugh; "Someone with the same sense of humour and a lovely smile," is more likely to bring a satisfying outcome.

Listen and watch for the outcome while you get on with life. Remember to suspend all judgement, and realise that repeating requests endlessly suggests you have not pressed the button hard enough first time. You have! So don't go chasing after your request, release it gladly and it will float towards you at the perfect time in the perfect way. If we ask, and then let go of *everything,* what is for us will come back to us.

Act in faith. Pure faith is hard to sustain, especially as our five senses constantly feed data to tell us, show us, and plug us into a reality that so often wants to argue. So, in order to keep the faith with this process where our grosser senses would mislead, keep a focus on how you feel, and keep reorientating to the peaceful heart-centre that knows we are always heard, understood and loved.

Say thank you and express gratitude for all the good things in your life – all the miracles! – that are already part of you, and that already help you to enjoy your creative processes. If in doubt, express thanks, and let gratitude flood out fear. Release fears that crop up, and keep living the best you can, inching forward.

As we become accustomed to clearing out our emotional baggage, releasing fear and negativity, suspending all judgement and acting in faith, answers do arrive more quickly and easily. With every success we understand more about how our personal creative power works. There is no such thing as a 'small' miracle. All expressions of love – all miracles – are maximal (9). Working with our own unique gifts and strengths, we naturally modify universal techniques for ourselves, while consciously releasing negativity, asking clearly for what we want and expressing gratitude, has immense value in itself. Master the art of living in the present, and honestly, it hardly matters then whether miracles show up: we simply enjoy our lives so much more, which is the best motivation in the world.

WHY BOTHER?

So now you have all the tools to make miracles. That's nice. I can stop writing, can I? Before we head off into the sunset, may I offer a few words of caution? There are an awful lot of cynics out there longing to tear down your optimism, yearning to make you see sense and tell you, "Don't waste your time with all that nonsense."

Taking too long to find answers to that annoying question, "Why?" has made for an uncomfortable life. Spirit would laugh here and say, "Yes, that's because you like to think you can do everything all alone and that listening to us is a sign of weakness. You have refused to accept help from anyone until you were utterly desperate." And they would be right. It has been like sitting on a pin-cushion. Remember those? The things we made in Primary One that looked like squashed hedgehogs, with pins and needles sticking up all over...

There is still some part of me that cannot rest until I have looked at every conceivable permutation of every question or difficulty. To say I am over-analytical would be a relaxed assessment. "Why?" never comes alone, but drags along its deflating pal, "What's the point?" But please don't ask me these questions, because then you will then be making it my job to tell you your answers. Instead, please start listening to yourself.

First we wait and listen. If we get into the habit of staying centred and returning to feelings of joy and bliss, refusing to be derailed by external demands or expectations, increasingly our joy reveals answers that feel right for us. Even the smallest steps are taken care of. The plumber may come to replace my heating system on Wednesday, when I "just happen" to be available. The doorbell rings and it is someone I was thinking about. A letter arrives that fills me with hope. I can ask, "What would you like me to know?" and answers and clarity will arrive, so long as I remain calm, relaxed and clear about the value of my joy.

All the time while we chase around doing stuff, comparing our lives to others and striving after bigger, better and best, we have been missing a central truth: our best lives are unfolding here, at the heart of our knowing, right now. When we are peaceful with ourselves and can ask for what we truly desire, the Universe can go into a high gear and bring us answers quickly.

The Universe is happy feeling our uniqueness. Our feelings and experiences are uniquely *us*. I can feel my joy. I may have recently been sorrowful or angry. Are you anguished? Make it a pure anguish that streams out of you and is earthed in the ground, where it can do no damage and leaves quickly, so that you feel refreshed and freer.

When we are being ourselves, our actions stem from a purer enjoyment and are far more likely to bring results that fit with what we truly choose. The point of living is to be ourselves, to the best and fullest extent that we can be. How does life feel when it works with us, instead of against us? That is where we are going. Before our minds really "understand" what is happening – and analyse it to death – we are suddenly joyful and successful creators, as Life intends us to be.

I am a tiny particle of the big world. But I am a particle! I am here. We ask, "Is there anybody out there?" We look outside, up there in the heavens above us for answers, our heads craning over the fence, past the horizon, into next week, next year, the next solar system. Like the next miracle cure on the shelves at the chemist's shop: over there, up yonder, always *somewhere else.*

Let's try looking right here for a change, at our feet, our shoes, at our hands. Which is easier for me now? Would I rather wait for Sputnik Twelve to bring back samples of life on Mars in an airtight plastic bag, or would I prefer to look for miracles closer to home? Hands up, who would choose the easy option? Me! Me! Yes, well, have you looked in the mirror? In ourselves, we can witness many miracles. The horizon over the next hill will keep. First, we can begin to see that the biggest miracle starts inside ourselves. Go within, because that is the birthplace of miracles.

As we expand our awareness we can listen politely to those many others who tell us that God, or peace, or love, or success lie somewhere else, around the next bend or into next month, or even within the next Nintendo Wii. Then we can carry on doing our own thing, knowing what we know and increasingly fine-tuning our understanding. We can ignore the diehards who insist that our experiences are improbable or our belief systems are facile. If you listen to what you know, your inner compass can tell you where to go and what to do.

You have the techniques you can deploy to see and experience the miracles that are already here, wrapping themselves around your life. After you have seen a few, you can make our own. If you have got any ideas from what is written here, you are well on the way to making your life more authentic.

The journey is a long one, so whenever we feel faint-hearted, it helps to remember…

You are precious

Presumably, you started reading this book because you have questions – about life, the Universe, this whole "being" thing. Existential crises are what I do best. Welcome, brother, sister, friend. We are all the same, down here. You think I don't know that? Why do you think I write this stuff? So that I can spell it out for myself again and again. I use my writing to teach myself. I am a very slow learner, though perhaps there is no hurry after all and the investment is worthwhile.

Results may be slow in coming and even on the best days, there seem to be unexpected setbacks, but I persist because I have this foolish idea that I am worth it, because I am: because I am here, because I am breathing. Because I came here to do this whole "life" thing as best I could. I came here, as we all did, prompted by a desire to show that living can be fun; and to learn how to put my desires in train despite all the cynics out there who might wonder at the lengths I go to; and despite apparent "difficulties" which would make it far easier for me to do nothing.

To put it another way, I love myself, therefore…I eat healthy and delicious food, I smile and laugh, I allow myself to receive goodness – because I believe in miracles. And I do everything I do simply because, whether I remember it or not, I am worthwhile. My small, fractured body is worthwhile. I repeat this one million times until I start to believe it. Conviction grows imperceptibly into truth, until one day – one magical day! – we *know* that what we have believed is totally true.

Like me, you can and will uncover inspiration that makes you cry; and at the same time you may come to gentle awareness that there is work still to do on self-love. (10) It is in loving ourselves as completely as we can, that we accord ourselves the respect we deserve, find our internal power and accept that we are deliberate creators of our lives.

Don't think about it

My husband asks me a question like, "Is it true that if something tastes disgusting, it's good for you?" and without pausing, I answer, "Yes, I'm sure! Well…I think so." Isn't it interesting, that every time we say, "I think so," we are actually expressing a sort of doubt? "Yes, I *think* so…" Yet, we pride ourselves on the brilliance of our thought processes. If our brains are so reliable, why do we constantly import doubt when we think? Instead, stop thinking about it. Resist the urge to analyse, refute, answer, agonize and dissect. Mental analysis does not work very well.

If you start thinking, you will bully yourself into giving up on all this positive stuff. Without being consciously aware, when we start to think about what we are doing here, we are bringing along our own inescapable element of doubt so that our hopes wilt and die. Resist the urge to douse cold water on your hopes with that modern mantra, the answer to all wonderful happenings and coincidence brave enough to show itself, "But that is incredible. I don't believe it!"

Many of your friends, too, will be more than happy to add their favourite arguments until you see sense again. After all, they will console, even the most cursory examination of the facts proves that all this miracle mumbo jumbo is completely unfounded, unscientific, unproven and therefore entirely use-less, pointless and deluded. We had better stick to reality. Grow up. Stop being so gullible. Our minds, which are so good at solving crossword puzzles and building boats and salvaging the best from a joint of meat, take upon themselves tasks which fit it less comfortably, less easily. Given its lead, the mind will tend to apply the brakes, or bully us away from our happiness.

Do yourself a favour and at the very least, reserve judgement until you see some results for yourself; until you have devised your own system of requests and gratitude that, despite resistance, incredulity and the busyness of life, seems to be making you feel better, more in touch with your deeper self, more willing to work hard at something or overlook the many stresses of daily life.

If you start to believe what you see, then wait. Wait and see and keep going with the positive belief in the meantime.

Don't talk about it

During my perusal of many books with a religious flavour, I have encountered the warning repeatedly offered by Jesus to any person he was curing: Go home and *do not talk about this* with your friends. Go quietly on your way and keep your own counsel. I have wondered why. As with most puzzles, it intrigued me until I started having a few coincidences and small miracles of my own.

The reason to rest peaceful for a while with what we discover is that in talking about wonderful things that happen to us, we are likely to encounter a wall of disbelief and gentle mockery that will shake at our new faith and loosen it. That reintroduction of cynicism into our new, fresh optimism which nourishes all miracles is what Jesus was warning against. Keep cynicism fenced off until the faith that is essential for healing has taken root and is firmly enough established to withstand a bit of withering scorn.

Developments in quantum physics are interesting, as is any study of the space-time continuum, the theory of relativity, the behaviour of light particles and so forth. Strangely, this vanguard of physics and of rational scientific exploration is now rediscovering that the wisdom of sages through the ages has more than a grain of truth in it. Now, we are beginning to understand that what wise listeners have been telling us for thousands of years about the nature of matter, the nature of creation and the meaning of time, might have been true all along: mind does influence matter. Your thoughts do create your present and your future. Time has a flexible quantity, which is influenced by our thoughts; and the world does indeed rearrange itself to deliver to us what we expect.

We have come full circle. We have travelled all the way around the block, past the "dark ages", through the Renaissance, past the philosophers of the En-lightenment. We have taken lots of wrong turns and made many fantastic scientific discoveries. We even have a brand new and hugely expensive particle accelerator which we hope will teach us something Earth-shattering about the nature of matter in the Universe.

And all this time the truth has been waiting for us, whispering, "I am the great I AM – and so are you. Go within and there will you find all your miracles. Go within." Tune in to your in-tuition, to what your inner wisdom can teach you. Don't take my word for it, go and find this out for yourself. You can do it.

While all living creatures are busy living and being their own particle accelerators, we all get signs, hints and nudges, to reassure us, or to make us stop and wonder whether this is really where we should be going! If your path is littered with difficulties, perhaps it is time to stand back and have another look. When the way is smooth and you don't have to think about it, you are on course. You have arrived. From that feeling comes all the right results.

Don't worry about it

Worrying repels happiness. When you worry you send out negative energy, which powerfully attracts to you the very thing you say you don't want. Worry energy is still energy and whatever you focus your energy on, whatever energy you deploy, pulls IT towards you. As Spirit tell me repeatedly, "Worrying doesn't help!" So try smiling instead. If you are tempted to take a dip down into your problems, raise your aim and deliberately look to something beyond, anything more pleasurable. Resist the urge to take a gander down sad memory lane and keep your focus on your present. What will your present be now, to yourself?

HOW DO YOU FEEL?

I have to ask you, how do you feel about this? Are you feeling a bit goofy because you wasted money on this book? Do you wish you had never started out on this quest because nothing seems to be working? Or are you happier and more optimistic than you expected to be?

Our feelings are our inner compass. Our natural, inherent emotions will keep us on the right track, if we can allow them to surface and get past all the external parts of our lives that we think make us happy or miserable. It can take a while for our relaxed selves – which we have spent so many years suppressing and shaping to expectations – to come out and blossom. It can take a while until we trust our feelings again. But they are our truth tellers, whispering at night and sending us dreams to read and heed.

I can imagine how you might feel if you meet up with friends or family and someone asks, "So, what are you reading at the moment?" You may mumble, change the subject or leave the room in a hurry. There is no point in making ourselves a laughing stock, after all. But now that my faith has taken hold and is more firmly rooted, I have the perfect answers to all my friendly cynics; to all those people who would prefer to douse cold water on smiling, singing and on optimism in general. Quite simply:

~ We need all the happiness we can get.

~ I am a nicer person when I feel happy.

~ Life is a miracle and we are all part of that miracle.

~ I feel peaceful when I read this sort of thing.

~ I feel authentic again.

~ I enjoy my own power.

~ My power refreshes and uplifts me.

If you meet more hostility than usual, you may gently suggest to those who firmly believe that all life is hard graft and difficulty, that their beliefs seem a bit heavy. With a bit of humour you might throw in the comment that you have reached an age where you don't mind being deluded and your critics can judge any book by the effect it has on you and on them.

We had better not say outright that people who are angst-ridden and fearful don't seem well served by their beliefs. They don't seem very happy… We had better not tell everyone that there is another way and that there is no need for constantly painful taboos and the sorrow that shrouds our lives and our deaths, because to tell them all this would not make the cynics happy. Many of us nurse our ailments like talismans. We think that our illnesses make us what we are, instead of seeing them as the barbs in a body that will respond better with sincere love and affection.

The body is the outer casing, the home for Spirit which lives here a while and likes to flex its creative muscles. When we listen to our intuition, to our guidance, we can achieve great things. Time is the buffer zone between the intentions we express, the choices we make and the outcomes we are looking for. Sooner or later, cynics will discover all this for themselves.

I find that the quest for miracles, for peace and happiness can be intensely lonely. Very few others actually believe me when I say that there is nothing to worry about. When I suggest that optimism is better than realism, when I suggest that the heaviness of this world is an illusion, I feel a weight of sorrow hovering at my back, keen to prove me wrong. Yet, I know that we all originate with the light, as does everything that comes to us.

In a dream about letting go of the old, releasing my fear of disapproval, I am sitting in an empty room. Someone has quit my side, unhappy with the way I am going, someone from the old days, who wants me to be as I have always been. But I have changed and cannot agree to do what they want, so they leave me. I feel abandoned and lost but I will not change my mind. I don't get up and run back to be with them. Instead, I sit on my own for a while until gradually, imperceptibly, the room fills with people all chatting happily to each other. All have come to be with me and with each other. In the end, the room is filled with interesting people. So – don't let fear of disapproval hold you back! Keep the faith!

Whatever happens, we will not stop shining our light. Sometimes it shines brightly and at other times it is dimmed by our preoccupation with worldly concerns. Our brightness is never extinguished, though; and I know that whatever brightens us and makes us fizz with excitement is intended to bless us. Excitement tells us something important, and with it, we reaffirm what we believe and see signs everywhere that we are on the right track. Chance meetings and opportunities are perfectly placed, so that life becomes meaningful and enjoyable; and all because we stop trying so hard.

I cannot listen all the time: I have many things to do. Even so, gradually more is revealed at a pace that makes learning both energizing and liberating. More is understood. I am happy. I am free. You can be too.

CROSSING THE LINE

We live divided lives. On the one hand, we know that we are inherently beautiful, lovely, powerful and connected to life. Children know this, without having it explained to them. When we reconnect with our deeper selves, we remember that we are part of a grand, joyful conspiracy of light on Earth, in a game that never ceases.

On the other hand, we create and then dwell within complicated lives that seem to demand so much of our energy. A great deal of thought and time is invested in defining ourselves in the world and in establishing and maintaining our position and guarding our possessions: so many locks, keys and passwords! We strive, we work and occasionally, we rest. What are we resting from? Why are we taking more holidays away from home than ever before? Perhaps because our everyday lives have become harshly and relentlessly structured to keep us away from peace and restful dreaming, so frenetic that we have to run and hide away on remote islands where there is no mobile signal, before we can switch off. And no sooner have we got settled on a beach with a towel and a water bottle than that irritating mind chatter starts up.

Wherever we are and whatever we are doing, the peace we are searching for can be found within. Within ourselves we can locate and strengthen the knowledge that we are safe, beautiful, cared for, loved and gentle. Increasingly, that light of knowing brightens our path and shows the way. As we dwell in peace and our light brightens, increasingly "bad" or "troublesome" situations resolve themselves or avoid us, while a better life flowers around us. Within the silence, at our heart, we can find the answers we are searching for to live authentically; while surrounded by our routines and our "must do" lists, our difficult working lives, gradually we become the controller of them, not ruled by them. Imperceptibly, as we open ourselves to the wisdom found in silence, we notice that we can stay there and be peaceful, whatever we are doing and even, and especially, when we have to engage with the world's processes and timetables.

To know that we are undertaking a transition from mind-based preoccupations to heart-centred lightness is to cross the thin line that divides our awareness between doing and having and simply being. Increasingly, as we enjoy refreshing feelings of staying present and alert to the power that pulses through our bodies, we allow growing certainty and joy to strengthen us.

Resistance to our quest for deeper peace is never far behind. To the ego, silence and presence spell its death; so the ego and its ceaseless mind chatter will fight with all its weapons – guilt, anger, feelings of hopelessness and overwhelm, futility, anxiety and self-loathing – to reacquaint us with the reality of the world and its grave preoccupations. It will fight me and make my body ache, cause me to have accidents and will retrieve from my memory long-lost grievances and fears that grip, take me back, shake my new composure and which *feel so real.*

Resistance is a pain, quite literally, but it is also a good sign that we are making real progress, rather than simply paying lip service to new ideas. *Any* increase in our awareness, however slight, is beneficial and is never lost in later setbacks we encounter. Increasing awareness is a one-way street to a better life, a positive feedback loop with truly transformative power. So we have a lot to gain from persisting with our hopes for a deeper, calmer and clearer future. Who on earth does not seek for certainty, peace, gentleness and love?

Here is a waking dream I had recently.

I am sitting on a tree stump in a corral, which is dry, dusty and arid. Red earth, with nothing growing in the space around me. I have been sitting here so long, I can hardly move. My beautiful little child comes through the fence gate and takes my hand. Thus we leave. I have no fear of getting lost in the lush, beautiful forests that surround us, because they are so beautiful and we can navigate by the stars on this crystal clear night. Wherever we walk, the path reveals itself, smooth and easy, beneath the trees. There is no fear of getting lost now because my child is with me, to keep me company and there are lots of delightful new things to see and places to go. There are places to rest and be peaceful.

As I walk, my shoes change for comfortable ones and my clothes alter too. I forget about the place I sat alone before, which is swallowed up by the forest and gradually reclaimed and regrown. I can leave it forever now, relax and walk, run or stride as I please. This forest is my home and any feelings of isolation are from the past. Gone and forgotten. Here in a forest of possibilities, I find a life of infinite beauty, variety, consolation, freedom and refreshment.

In doing what we enjoy – both alone and in the company of others – things work out easily and quickly. The more we notice and believe this, the more exciting life becomes: life rejoices to have found other souls who are listening and learning to take heed. When we take the careful route that we are led to – instead of arguing – Life works for us as it is meant to. The results can be so beautiful.

NOTES

1) The Gospel of Matthew 25:29

2) *A Course in Miracles,* p 31, 2nd ed.
    Viking Penguin, 1996

3) *Why Forgive?* Johann Christoph Arnold,
    Plough Publishing House, 2010

4) *Collins English Dictionary,* HarperCollins
    Publishers, 3rd Ed. 1995

5) The *Writers' and Artists' Yearbook,*
    Bloomsbury Yearbooks

6) Abraham/Hicks, *Ask and It is Given:*
    Learning to Manifest the Laws of Attraction,
    Hay House, 2004

7) The Gospel of Matthew 19.24

8) Neale Donald Walsch, *Conversations with*
    God, volume 3, p 257 Hampton Roads
    Publishing Company, 2003

9) *A Course in Miracles*, p 3

10) Louise Hay, *You Can Heal Your Life,*
    Hay House Publishing, 1984

ABOUT FRAN MACILVEY

Fran was born in Congo in 1965 and spent eight years at boarding school in Scotland. She gained honours in Scots law and worked as a solicitor for ten years before turning to her first love, writing. Her memoir, *Trapped: My Life with Cerebral Palsy* (Skyhorse Publishing (2014/2016, ISBN: 9781510704121) is an Amazon international bestseller.

Fran's second book, *Happiness Matters* (ISBN: 9781999713607) and *Making Miracles* explore how we can all find more happiness and fulfilment in life – what Fran calls, "gleaning something valuable from forty years of making mistakes." If you have enjoyed reading *Making Miracles* please consider writing a review.

Fran is currently writing a series of novels about women in the law. In her spare time she reads, swims, blogs, rides a lovely horse called Mr Bob, sings in the shower and dances where no-one can see her.

If you would like to contact Fran, please email franmacilvey@fastmail.com or get in touch at

https://www.franmacilvey.com.

Thanks...

My sincerest thanks to...all my followers, readers and on-line colleagues, and in particular, Bernie Leslie, Catherine Lenderi, Cherry Gregory, literary consultant Claire Wingfield, David Price, Diana Noel-Paton and everyone at The Thistle Foundation, Diane Dickson, Dilek Taylor, Dorothy Chitty, Doug Simpson, Elouise Renich Fraser, Emma Crees, Fiona Bennett, Fleur, John and Dolly Boyle, Frank Kusy, Jane Ambrose, Jane Dixon-Smith, Jane Risdon, Janet Hughes, Jerry Waxler, John Bayliss, John and Kerstin Phillips, Joy Godfrey, Judy Adams, Julie D'Amour, Karen Concannon, Lucinda E Clarke, Majk Stokes, Malcolm Scullion, Margaret Skea, Michael McEwan, Michèle and Andrew Alter Brenton, Patti Tingen, Rachael Cloughton, Rose Ann Fraser Ritchie, Shannon Page, Valerie Poore.

9 781999 713621